EAVDI YEARBOOK 2015

REVIEWS IN VETERINARY DIAGNOSTIC IMAGING

EUROPEAN ASSOCIATION OF VETERINARY DIAGNOSTIC IMAGING, LTD

EAVDI Yearbook Editorial Board 2015

Regine Hagen
Sandra Martig
Mary-Elizabeth Raw
Allison Zwingenberger

Prepared for publishing by

Mike French

EAVDI Officers 2015

President

Markus Tassani-Prell
Tierklinik Hofheim
Im Langgewann 9
D-65719 Hofheim am Taunus
GERMANY
Tel: 0049-(0)6192-290290
Fax: 0049-(0)6192-290299
president@eavdi.org

Secretary

Valentina Piola
V. Tito Groppo 13/7
16043 Chiavari (Ge)-Italy
Tel +39 328 2494322
secretary@eavdi.org

Treasurer

Anna Groth
North Downs Specialist Referrals
The Friesian Building 3&4
The Dairy Brewerstreet Business Park
Surrey RH1 4QP
UK
treasurer@eavdi.org

Web Editor

Mat Hennessey
webeditor@eavdi.org

CONTENTS

Introduction   vii

1 Advanced Neuroimaging in Veterinary Science   1

   Philippa J. Johnson

2 Image-Guided Radiotherapy: Principles and Applications in
   Veterinary Medicine   15

   Carla Rohrer Bley

3 Diagnostic Imaging of the Equine Back   25

   Fabrice Audigié, Virginie Coudry, Sandrine Jacquet, Lélia Bertoni,
   Jean-Marie Denoix

4 From Quantitative to Nano-computed Tomography:
   Research and Clinical Applications   47

   Sandra Martig

5 Low-field Magnetic Resonance Imaging of the Canine Stifle
   Joint   63

   Martin Konar

6 Small Intestinal Ultrasonography in Dogs and Cats   93

   Lorrie Gaschen and Alexandre LeRoux

7 Abstracts From German Publications 2014 and Early 2015   105

   Abstracts selected and edited by Sandra Martig

INTRODUCTION

The 2015 EAVDI yearbook is a collection of review papers of outstanding quality. Experts from different institutions explain the details of their work using state of the art equipment. This information is very useful for residents in diagnostic imaging, for other specialists as well as for practitioners.

Specialisation in veterinary medicine is continuing to progress, and a large body of research abstracts are available in journals and presentations covering all aspects of diagnostic imaging. In addition to this exploration of details, it is necessary to get practical and clinically relevant information at the same time.

The authors of this yearbook, Philippa J. Johnson, Carla Rohrer Bley, Fabrice Audigié and his team, Sandra Martig, Martin Konar and Lorrie Gaschen together with Alexandre LeRoux did an excellent job. They have provided us with review articles combining general and brand-new information. A collection of German abstracts selected and edited by Sandra Martig makes this yearbook complete.

It was a great pleasure to read these articles, and I´m looking forward to the next EAVDI yearbook.

Many thanks to the authors and to the editors, Allison Zwingenberger, Sandra Martig, Regine Hagen and Mary-Elizabeth Raw.

Markus Tassani-Prell, EAVDI President

1 ADVANCED NEUROIMAGING IN VETERINARY SCIENCE

Philippa J. Johnson

Institute of Psychiatry, Psychology and Neuroscience, Kings College London, UK

Introduction

Advances in magnetic resonance imaging (MRI) have taken place rapidly in the last twenty years with the development of a number of new techniques to assess not only the structure of the brain but also its function, connectivity, plasticity, diffusion and biochemical properties. Currently, the majority of MRI techniques used in veterinary neurology revolve around structural MRI sequences. With greater access to higher powered MRI systems in university veterinary hospitals and veterinary collaboration with neuroscientists, computer scientists, medical physicists and human neuroradiologists, some of these newer techniques are starting to be published in the veterinary literature. In this essay I will discuss the basic methodology behind the techniques of diffusion weighted imaging (DWI), diffusion tensor imaging (DTI), magnetic resonance spectroscopy (MRS) and functional magnetic resonance imaging (fMRI) and provide a current literature review for each.

Abbreviations

ADCs	Apparent diffusion coefficients
BOLD	Blood oxygen level dependent contrast
DTI	Diffusion tensor imaging
DWI	Diffusion weighted imaging
FA	Fractional anisotropy
fMRI	Functional magnetic resonance imaging
MD	Mean diffusivity
MRI	Magnetic resonance imaging
MRS	Magnetic resonance spectroscopy
RGB	Red/green/blue

Diffusion Weighted Imaging

Magnetic resonance imaging relies on the resonating signal from hydrogen protons to form an image. This hydrogen is predominantly present within the water molecules of brain tissue. Diffusion imaging is able to detect the microscopic free movement of these water molecules. This data is used to calculate apparent diffusion coefficients (ADCs), which are quantitative measures of water movement within each voxel. These measures are displayed on ADC maps. The degree of water molecule diffusion present is dependent on the structure of the tissue and is altered when there is tissue damage.[1,2] The diffusion characteristics of the normal canine brain have been described and it was identified that there are significantly different ADCs between different regions of the brain. It has been suggested that this is due to alterations in myelination, neural density and fibre orientation within these regions.[3]

The diffusion characteristics of various brain pathologies, both in veterinary patients and in canine models for disease, have been described in the literature. Diffusion weighted imaging has been found to be valuable in the imaging of cerebrovascular accidents in veterinary patients. Diffusion is restricted in necrotic and compromised tissue affected by infarction. This results in these lesions being hyperintense on diffusion weighted images and hypointense on the calculated ADC maps (FIGURE 1).[4,5] Similar findings are described in humans where the restricted water molecule diffusion is thought to be due to the movement of water into damaged cells.[6] Canine models for stroke lesions have been developed to take advantage of these similarities between canine and human cerebrovascular lesions. Diffusion weighted sequences have been used extensively in these experimental dogs to monitor the effects of acute infarction and its evolution over time.[7-9]

Although ischemic infarction is the most clinically recognised indication for DWI, there is utility for the use of this technique in other pathologies. When the diffusion characteristics of inflammatory, neoplastic and cerebrovascular lesions were evaluated in clinical canine patients, water molecule diffusion was found to be restricted not only within acute non-haemorrhagic infarcts but also within meningiomas, glial cell tumours and granulomatous meningoencephalitis.[10]

Diffusion Tensor Imaging

Diffusion tensor imaging goes a step further than simply measuring the diffusivity of water. It is able to measure the degree of diffusion along certain axes to calculate 3 eigenvalues (λ_1, λ_2, λ_3) and detect the orientation of the diffusion to form 3 eigenvectors (υ_1, υ_2, υ_3). When water diffusion is completely unrestricted, it diffuses randomly in all directions and the 3 eigenvalues are approximately equal; this is termed isotropic diffusion. When there is differential diffusion along one or another axes and the 3 eigenvalues are therefore

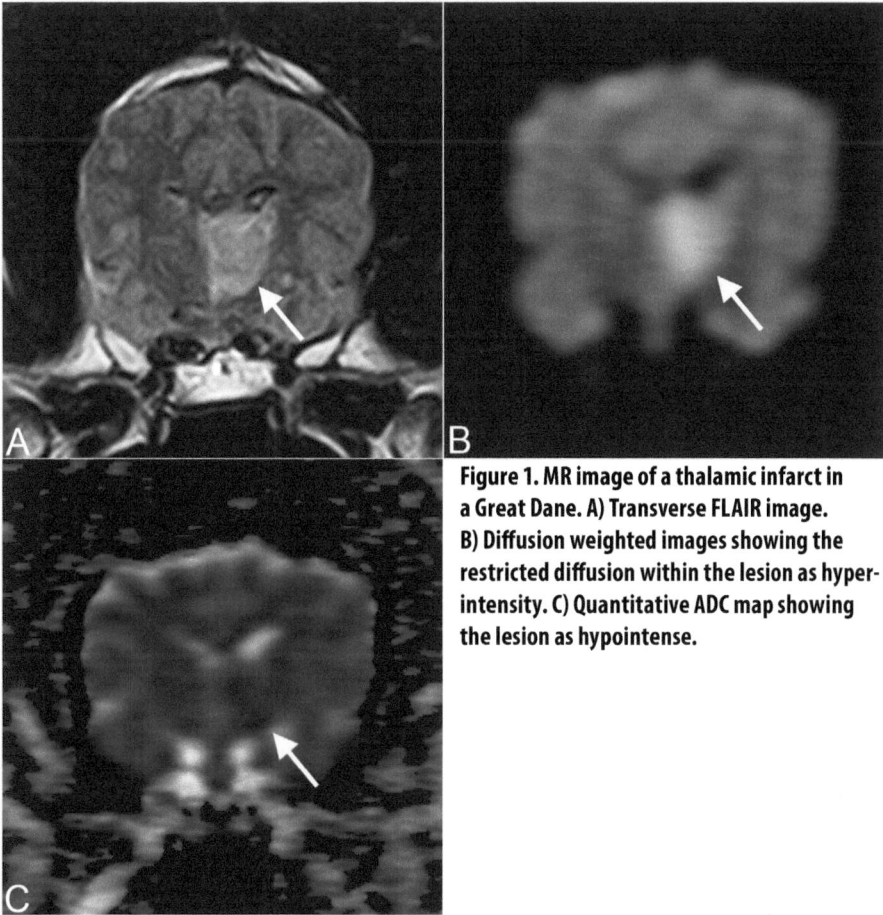

Figure 1. MR image of a thalamic infarct in a Great Dane. A) Transverse FLAIR image. B) Diffusion weighted images showing the restricted diffusion within the lesion as hyperintensity. C) Quantitative ADC map showing the lesion as hypointense.

not equal, then this is termed anisotropic diffusion (FIGURE 2). In different tissues the diffusion of water has different characteristics. For instance, in white matter tracts the diffusion of water molecules follows the line of the tract and therefore has markedly axial anisotropic diffusion, whereas in CSF the molecular diffusion is completely random and is therefore isotropic.[1,11]

These characteristics of diffusion can be used to form different types of brain maps. Mean diffusivity maps (MD maps) demonstrate the average mobility of the water molecules in each voxel (FIGURE 3A). Fractional anisotropy maps (FA maps), on the other hand, demonstrate the shape and degree of anisotropy of diffusion within each voxel (FIGURE 3B). From FA maps, red-green-blue (RGB) maps can be created using colours to show the direction of the diffusion (FIGURE 3C). These maps can provide information as to the organisation of white matter and improve our ability to evaluate tissue microstructure.[1]

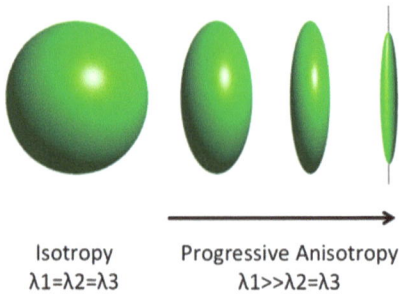

Isotropy
$\lambda1=\lambda2=\lambda3$

Progressive Anisotropy
$\lambda1>>\lambda2=\lambda3$

Figure 2. Different types of water molecule diffusion. Isotropic diffusion occurs when diffusion is completely random and unrestricted and all of the eigenvalues are equal. Anisotropic diffusion occurs when water molecule movement is restricted in certain planes and as a result the eigenvalues are not equal, with one being is greater than the others.

Diffusion tensor imaging is also the technology underlying the 3-D modelling technique of tractography. Tractography utilizes the concept that water diffusion along white matter is markedly anisotropic. This technique is therefore able to recreate the structure of the white matter tracts indirectly by assessing the anisotropic water diffusion along them. It identifies the primary eigenvector within each voxel and starting from a seed voxel propagates a 3-D curve, using the direction of the vectors to demonstrate the direction of the white matter pathway. This allows formation of 3D images demonstrating the structure of the white matter tracts. This technique correlates well with pathological specimens (FIGURE 4).[12]

Diffusion tensor imaging has been utilized in humans for anatomic studies and to identify white matter structural changes in both neurological and psychological diseases.[12] In dogs DTI of the normal spinal cord has been documented in dachshunds, beagles and in a mixed breed population.[13-15] Additionally the white matter tracts of the normal canine brain both *ex vivo* and *in vivo* have been mapped using DTI and tractography.[16,17] Post mortem studies on canine brains have found good correlation between 7T MRI DTI and histopathological dissection.[18,19] The effects of pathologies, including disc herniation, extradural fibrosarcoma, fibrocartilagenous embolism and myelomalacia, on the diffusion characteristics and tractography of the canine spinal cord have been published on a select number of cases.[15]

More work has been performed on cats in this field. The normal anatomical diffusion structure of the brain and spinal cord has been documented in cats in a number of studies.[20-23] Cats have also been utilized as experimental models for brain oedema and spinal cord injury. In experimentally induced brain oedema, FA was significantly decreased and remained decreased even after resolution.[24] Spinal cord imaging in cats can be affected by poor image quality; however, with optimization, DTI of spinal cord injury can demonstrate disruption to the fibre bundles and detect a significantly lower FA at the site of the lesion.[20,25] Neural development has been studied and longitudinally followed using diffusion tensor techniques in both dogs and cats.[26,27]

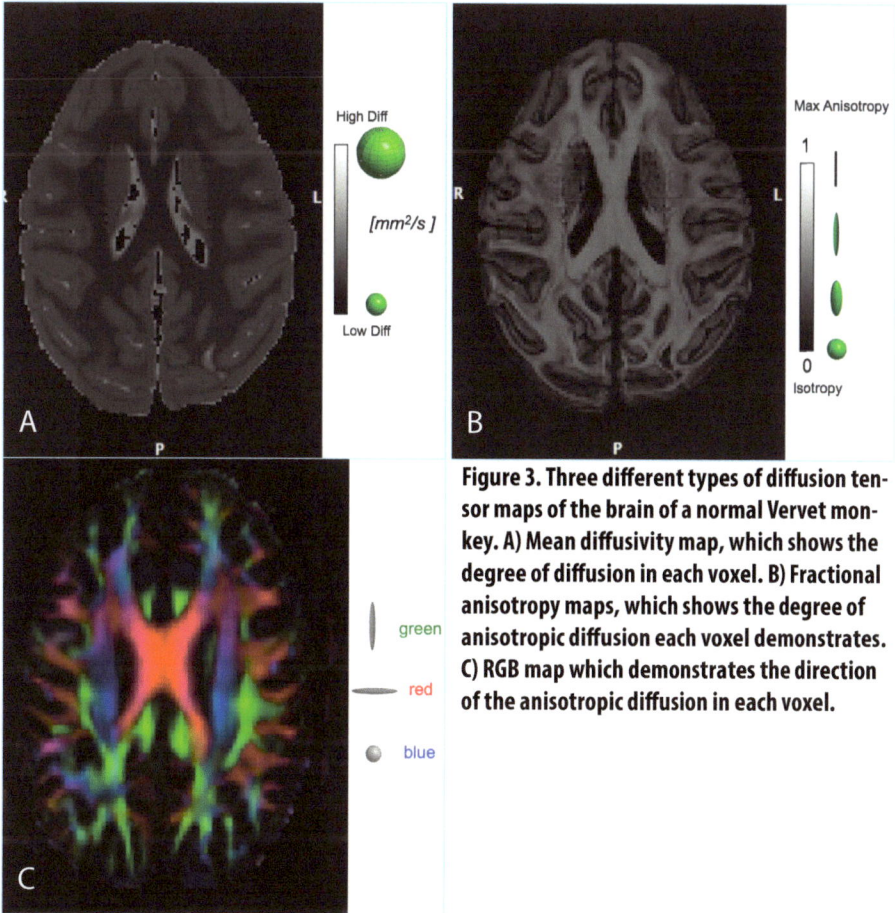

Figure 3. Three different types of diffusion tensor maps of the brain of a normal Vervet monkey. A) Mean diffusivity map, which shows the degree of diffusion in each voxel. B) Fractional anisotropy maps, which shows the degree of anisotropic diffusion each voxel demonstrates. C) RGB map which demonstrates the direction of the anisotropic diffusion in each voxel.

Magnetic Resonance Spectroscopy

Magnetic resonance spectroscopy is able to detect the different resonating frequencies associated with different metabolites. The molecular structure of each metabolite is composed of a benzene ring, which is bound to various configurations of hydrogen and other ions. The resonant frequency of the ions is altered by their interaction with the benzene ring. This is due to the fact that the benzene ring forms a separate magnetic field, which alters the magnetization of the protons and thus changes the overall resonant frequency of the molecule. The magnitude of the signal at these different frequencies can be detected and displayed on a spectrum, with each frequency spike representing the concentration of each metabolite. In the brain, there are specific metabolites that can provide biochemical information about the tissue itself. The specific metabolites that are detectable with MRS, their resonant frequency and biochemical functional correlates are listed in Table 1.[28-30]

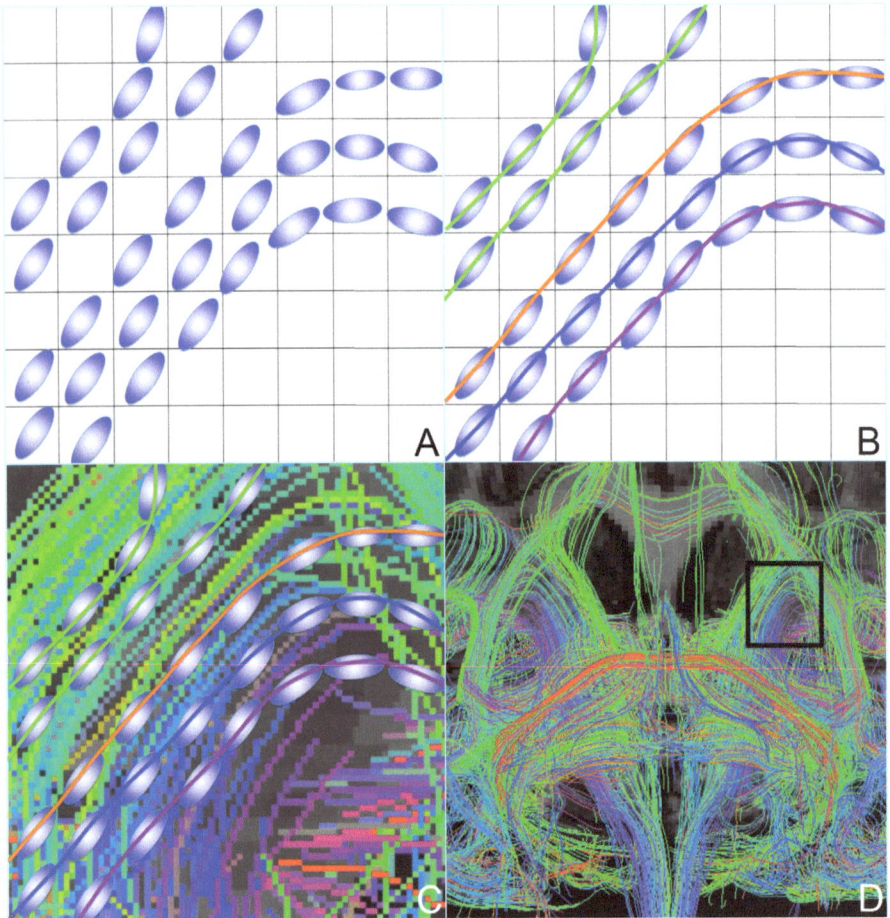

Figure 4. Eigenvectors are utilized to map out the path of white matter tracts in tractography. A) The anisotropic water diffusion in each voxel is detected. B) The principal eigenvector of the diffusion is used to track a line from voxel to voxel consistent with the tract of the white matter. C) The tracts are overlayed onto a real tractography image. D) Ventral view of the whole brain tractography of a Vervet monkey. The black square demonstrates the extract used in image C.

The technique of ^{1}H MRS at 3T has been optimized in canine cadavers and applied to multiple brain regions in healthy beagles using a long echo time multivoxel technique.[31,32] Additionally, protocols and standard metabolite reference values have been published for a single-voxel, short echo time ^{1}H MRS 3T technique and a single voxel long echo time 1.5T ^{1}H MRS technique in healthy beagles (FIGURE 5A).[33,34]

Metabolite	Resonant Frequency (ppm)	Biochemical Function
N-acetyl aspartate (NAA)	2.02	Neuronal integrity
Choline (Cho)	3.10	Membrane synthesis and degradation
Creatinine (Cr)	3.00	Energy metabolism
Glutamate (Glu)	3.75	Neurotransmission excitation
Glutamine (Gln)	2.10-2.50	Neurotransmission regulation
Myoinositol (MI)	3.52	Intracellular second messenger system
Lactate (Lac)	1.33	Anaerobic glycolysis and only observed in the brain with brain ischaemia

Table 1. Metabolites that are detectable with MRS, their resonant frequency in parts per million (ppm) and their markers for biochemical functional correlates.

The ^{1}H MRS technique is able to detect alterations in these metabolites in a number of disease processes in veterinary patients, including inflammatory brain disease, neoplasia and hepatic encephalopathy (FIGURE 5B).[35-37] The disruption of metabolite concentrations is significantly different between inflammatory and neoplastic lesions, helping to differentiate these conditions. However, when trying to use ^{1}H MRS for the differentiation of tumour types in the canine brain, the metabolite changes were too similar between meningioma and glioma to form useful diagnostic criteria.[37]

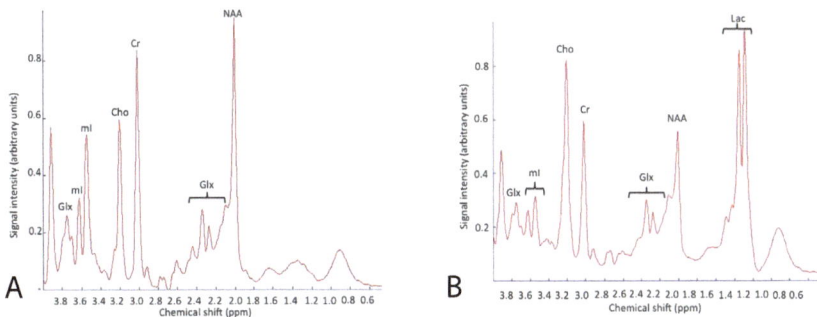

Figure 5. MR spectroscopy figures from two dogs. These spectra demonstrate peaks that include N-acetyl aspartate (NAA), choline (Cho), creatinine (Cr), glutamate (Glu), glutamine (Gln) myoinositol (MI) and lactate (Lac). A) A healthy beagle spectrum demonstrating the spikes of each metabolite within the normal brain. B) A spectrum taken from a brain with granulomatous meningo-encephalitis. There is a reduction in NAA and Cr and an increase in Cho. There is also a large spike of lactate, which is only present in the brain when there is anaerobic glycolysis occurring. Images courtesy of Dr. Ines Carrera.

Functional Magnetic Resonance Imaging

Functional magnetic resonance imaging utilizes the concept that with neuronal stimulation there is an associated increase in oxygenated blood flow to that region of neural tissue.[38] Detection of this increased regional blood flow enables identification of regions of increased neuronal activity. Oxygenated blood has an altered magnetization when compared to deoxygenated blood due to the effects of oxygen binding to haemoglobin.[39] This variable magnetization of haemoglobin results in oxygenated blood having altered signal characteristics on MRI when compared to deoxygenated blood. From this concept, blood oxygen level-dependent (BOLD) contrast was developed, allowing MRI to detect neuronal activation in the brain.[40]

Functional MRI has been utilized extensively in human neurological and psychological research and optimally requires the participant to be conscious. In dogs, both anaesthetized and conscious studies have been performed, whereas only anaesthetized studies have been performed in cats. Anaesthesia has an overall effect on cerebral blood flow and thus BOLD signal; however, it has been found that in dogs the BOLD response is similar between different anaesthetic protocol types and dosages.[41]

Most fMRI studies require some form of stimulus to be applied at a specific time to allow for differences in BOLD signal between control and stimulus time frames to be identified. In anaesthetized animals the effects of visual stimulus on activation of the visual neural system has been evaluated in both dogs and cats. In dogs, this has provided more information about the visual neural pathway and effects of monocular and binocular stimulation.[42] In cats, fMRI has been combined with 3D DTI to further characterize the functional and axonal connectivity of the visual cortex.[43]

The concept of performing fMRI on conscious dogs has been described. Dogs were acclimatised to the noise of the MRI and trained to lie motionless within the scanner during acquisition (FIGURE 6).[44] Acceptable motion levels were achieved and visible neural responses to stimuli were observed. Reward stimulus has been evaluated in a number of studies. Neural activation has been detected in response to reward stimulus.[44,45] When reward stimulus was given in different forms (by a familiar human, an unfamiliar human and a computer screen) the degree of neural response observed appeared to correlate to dog temperament.[46] Voice stimuli have also been utilized in conscious dogs and identified that not only did the auditory system show activation but also emotional valence-sensitive regions. This suggests that dogs, like humans, extract emotional information from voices.[47] When scent stimuli were evaluated in the conscious dog, it was found that although the olfactory bulb/peduncle activated similarly to scents from self, a familiar human, a strange human and a strange dog, the activation within the caudate nucleus, responsible for positive associations, was maximal when the dog smelt the familiar human.[48]

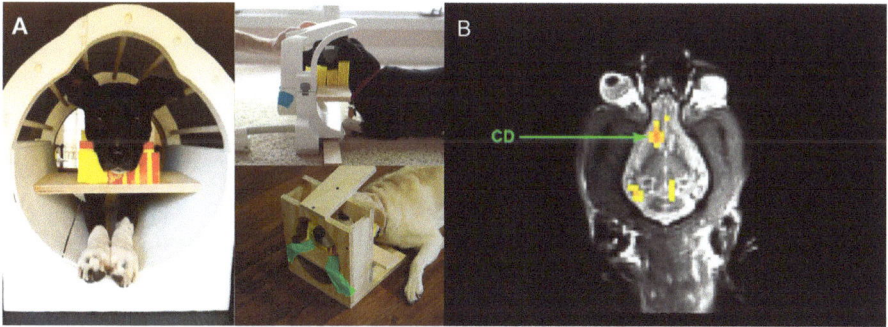

Figure 6. Functional MRI in conscious dogs. A) Training of the dogs with mock head coils and head rests to keep the head as motionless as possible. B) The statistical map of the combined results of two conscious fMRI scans and the brain activation to a reward stimulus. Activation present within the caudate nucleus (CD) is highlighted. Images adapted from published figures (https://creative-commons.org/licenses/by/4.0/legalcode).[44,45]

These advanced neuroimaging techniques require a high degree of technical skill, and the processing steps are still being developed for veterinary patients. However, there is significant potential for these advances to allow us to investigate the animal brain far more deeply. MRI is now not only telling us about the basic structure of the brain but is also able to provide biochemical information about the brain tissue, demonstrate the microstructure and connectivity of the white matter tracts and help us to further understand brain function in animals. The use of these techniques in the diagnosis of brain pathology has merely scratched the surface and in time may help improve diagnosis and provide increased prognostic information for owners without having to resort to invasive techniques.

References

1.   Johansen-Berg H, Behrens T. *Diffusion MRI: from quantitative measurement to in vivo neuroanatomy.* Academic Press, 2013.

2.   Neil JJ. Diffusion imaging concepts for clinicians. *J Magn Reson Imaging.* 2008;**27**:1-7.

3.   Hartmann A, Soffler C, Failing K, Schaubmar A, Kramer M, Schmidt MJ. Diffusion-weighted magnetic resonance imaging of the normal canine brain. *Vet Radiol Ultrasound.* 2014;**55**:592-598.

4.   Garosi L, McConnell JF, Platt SR, Barone G, Baron JC, de Lahunta A, et al. Clinical and topographic magnetic resonance characteristics of suspected brain infarction in 40 dogs. *J Vet Intern Med.* 2006;**20**:311-321.

5. McConnell JF, Garosi L, Platt SR. Magnetic resonance imaging findings of presumed cerebellar cerebrovascular accident in twelve dogs. *Vet Radiol Ultrasound*. 2005;**46**:1-10.

6. Schaefer PW, Grant PE, Gonzalez RG. Diffusion-weighted MR imaging of the brain. *Radiology*. 2000;**217**:331-345.

7. Harris AD, Kosior RK, Chen HS, Andersen LB, Frayne R. Evolution of hyperacute stroke over 6 hours using serial MR perfusion and diffusion maps. *J Magn Reson Imaging*. 2009;**29**:1262-1270.

8. Kang BT, Jang DP, Gu SH, Lee JH, Jung DI, Lim CY, et al. MRI features in a canine model of ischemic stroke: correlation between lesion volume and neurobehavioral status during the subacute stage. *Comp Med*. 2009;**59**:459-464.

9. Shaibani A, Khawar S, Shin W, Cashen TA, Schirf B, Rohany M, et al. First results in an MR imaging—compatible canine model of acute stroke. *Am J Neuroradiol*. 2006;**27**:1788-1793.

10. Sutherland-Smith J, King R, Faissler D, Ruthazer R, Sato A. Magnetic resonance imaging apparent diffusion coefficients for histologically confirmed intracranial lesions in dogs. *Vet Radiol Ultrasound*. 2011;**52**:142-148.

11. Basser PJ, Mattiello J, LeBihan D. MR diffusion tensor spectroscopy and imaging. *Biophys J*. 1994;**66**:259-267.

12. Dell'Acqua F, Catani M. Structural human brain networks: hot topics in diffusion tractography. *Curr Opin Neurol*. 2012;**25**:375-383.

13. Griffin JFt, Cohen ND, Young BD, Eichelberger BM, Padua A, Jr., Purdy D, et al. Thoracic and lumbar spinal cord diffusion tensor imaging in dogs. *J Magn Reson Imaging*. 2013;**37**:632-641.

14. Hobert MK, Stein VM, Dziallas P, Ludwig DC, Tipold A. Evaluation of normal appearing spinal cord by diffusion tensor imaging, fiber tracking, fractional anisotropy, and apparent diffusion coefficient measurement in 13 dogs. *Acta Vet Scand*. 2013;**55**:36.

15. Pease A, Miller R. The use of diffusion tensor imaging to evaluate the spinal cord in normal and abnormal dogs. *Vet Radiol Ultrasound*. 2011;**52**:492-497.

16. Anaya Garcia MS, Hernandez Anaya JS, Marrufo Melendez O, Velazquez Ramirez JL, Palacios Aguiar R. In vivo study of cerebral white matter in the dog using diffusion tensor tractography. *Vet Radiol Ultrasound*. 2015;**56**:188-195.

17. Jacqmot O, Van Thielen B, Fierens Y, Hammond M, Willekens I, Van Schuerbeek P, et al. Diffusion tensor imaging of white matter tracts in the dog brain. *Anat Rec*. 2013;**296**:340-349.

18. Pierce TT, Calabrese E, White LE, Chen SD, Platt SR, Provenzale JM. Segmentation of the canine corpus callosum using diffusion-tensor imaging tractography. *Am J Roentgenol.* 2014;**202**:W19-25.

19. Wei PT, Leong D, Calabrese E, White L, Pierce T, Platt S, et al. Diffusion tensor imaging of neural tissue organization: correlations between radiologic and histologic parameters. *Neuroradiol J.* 2013;**26**:501-510.

20. Cohen-Adad J, Benali H, Hoge RD, Rossignol S. In vivo DTI of the healthy and injured cat spinal cord at high spatial and angular resolution. *NeuroImage.* 2008;**40**:685-697.

21. Cohen-Adad J, Benali H, Rossignol S. Methodology for MR diffusion tensor imaging of the cat spinal cord. *Conf Proc IEEE Eng Med Biol Soc.* 2007;**2007**:323-326.

22. Ronen I, Kim KH, Garwood M, Ugurbil K, Kim DS. Conventional DTI vs. slow and fast diffusion tensors in cat visual cortex. *Magn Reson Med.* 2003;**49**:785-790.

23. Smith JM, James MF, Bockhorst KH, Smith MI, Bradley DP, Papadakis NG, et al. Investigation of feline brain anatomy for the detection of cortical spreading depression with magnetic resonance imaging. *J Anat.* 2001;**198**:537-554.

24. Zhao FY, Kuroiwa T, Miyasakai N, Tanabe F, Nagaoka T, Akimoto H, et al. Diffusion tensor feature in vasogenic brain edema in cats. *Acta Neurochir Suppl.* 2006;**96**:168-170.

25. Ellingson BM, Sulaiman O, Kurpad SN. High-resolution in vivo diffusion tensor imaging of the injured cat spinal cord using self-navigated, interleaved, variable-density spiral acquisition (SNAILS-DTI). *Magn Reson Imaging.* 2010;**28**:1353-1360.

26. Takahashi E, Dai G, Rosen GD, Wang R, Ohki K, Folkerth RD, et al. Developing neocortex organization and connectivity in cats revealed by direct correlation of diffusion tractography and histology. *Cereb Cortex.* 2011;**21**:200-211.

27. Wu YC, Field AS, Duncan ID, Samsonov AA, Kondo Y, Tudorascu D, et al. High b-value and diffusion tensor imaging in a canine model of dysmyelination and brain maturation. *NeuroImage.* 2011;**58**:829-837.

28. de Graaf RA. *In Vivo NMR Spectroscopy.* John Wiley & Sons, 2008.

29. Rae CD. A guide to the metabolic pathways and function of metabolites observed in human brain 1H magnetic resonance spectra. *Neurochem Res.* 2014;**39**:1-36.

30. Ross AJ, Sachdev PS. Magnetic resonance spectroscopy in cognitive research. *Brain Res Brain Res Rev.* 2004;**44**:83-102.

31. Ober CP, Warrington CD, Feeney DA, Jessen CR, Steward S. Optimizing a protocol for (1) H-magnetic resonance spectroscopy of the canine brain at 3T. *Vet Radiol Ultrasound*. 2013;**54**:149-158.

32. Warrington CD, Feeney DA, Ober CP, Jessen CR, Steward SM, Armien AG, et al. Relative metabolite concentrations and ratios determined by use of 3-T region-specific proton magnetic resonance spectroscopy of the brain of healthy Beagles. *Am J Vet Res*. 2013;**74**:1291-1303.

33. Carrera I, Richter H, Meier D, Kircher PR, Dennler M. Regional metabolite concentrations in the brain of healthy dogs measured by use of short echo time, single voxel proton magnetic resonance spectroscopy at 3.0 Tesla. *Am J Vet Res*. 2015;**76**:129-141.

34. Ono K, Kitagawa M, Ito D, Tanaka N, Watari T. Regional variations and age-related changes detected with magnetic resonance spectroscopy in the brain of healthy dogs. *Am J Vet Res*. 2014;**75**:179-186.

35. Beckmann K, Carrera I, Steffen F, Golini L, Kircher PR, Schneider U, et al. A newly designed radiation therapy protocol in combination with prednisolone as treatment for meningoencephalitis of unknown origin in dogs: a prospective pilot study introducing magnetic resonance spectroscopy as monitor tool. *Acta Vet Scand*. 2015;**57**:4.

36. Carrera I, Kircher PR, Meier D, Richter H, Beckman K, Dennler M. In vivo proton magnetic resonance spectroscopy for the evaluation of hepatic encephalopathy in dogs. *Am J Vet Res*. 2014;**75**:818-827.

37. Stadler KL, Ober CP, Feeney DA, Jessen CR. Multivoxel proton magnetic resonance spectroscopy of inflammatory and neoplastic lesions of the canine brain at 3.0 T. *Am J Vet Res*. 2014;**75**:982-989.

38. Roy CS, Sherrington CS. On the Regulation of the Blood-supply of the Brain. *J Physiol*. 1890;**11**:85-158 117.

39. Pauling L, Coryell CD. The magnetic properties and structure of hemoglobin, oxyhemoglobin and carbonmonoxyhemoglobin. *P Natl Acad Sci USA*, 1936;210-216.

40. Ogawa S, Lee TM, Kay AR, Tank DW. Brain magnetic resonance imaging with contrast dependent on blood oxygenation. *P Natl Acad Sci USA*. 1990;**87**:9868-9872.

41. Willis CK, Quinn RP, McDonell WM, Gati J, Parent J, Nicolle D. Functional MRI as a tool to assess vision in dogs: the optimal anesthetic. *Vet Ophthalmol*. 2001;**4**:243-253.

42. Willis CK, Quinn RP, McDonell WM, Gati J, Partlow G, Vilis T. Functional MRI activity in the thalamus and occipital cortex of anesthetized dogs induced by monocular and binocular stimulation. *Can J Vet Res*. 2001;**65**:188-195.

43. Kim DS, Kim M, Ronen I, Formisano E, Kim KH, Ugurbil K, et al. In vivo mapping of functional domains and axonal connectivity in cat visual cortex using magnetic resonance imaging. *Magn Reson Imaging*. 2003;**21**:1131-1140.

44. Berns GS, Brooks AM, Spivak M. Functional MRI in awake unrestrained dogs. *PLoS ONE*. 2012;7:e38027.

45. Berns GS, Brooks A, Spivak M. Replicability and heterogeneity of awake unrestrained canine FMRI responses. *PLoS ONE*. 2013;**8**:e81698.

46. Cook PF, Spivak M, Berns GS. One pair of hands is not like another: caudate BOLD response in dogs depends on signal source and canine temperament. *PeerJ*. 2014;**2**:e596.

47. Andics A, Gacsi M, Farago T, Kis A, Miklosi A. Voice-sensitive regions in the dog and human brain are revealed by comparative fMRI. *Curr Biol*. 2014;**24**:574-578.

48. Berns GS, Brooks AM, Spivak M. Scent of the familiar: an fMRI study of canine brain responses to familiar and unfamiliar human and dog odors. *Behav Processes*. 2015;**110**:37-46.

2 IMAGE-GUIDED RADIOTHERAPY: PRINCIPLES AND APPLICATIONS IN VETERINARY MEDICINE

Carla Rohrer Bley

Division of Radiation Oncology, Vetsuisse-Faculty, University of Zurich, Switzerland

Abbreviations	
CT	Computed tomography
IGRT	Image-guided radiotherapy
IMRT	Intensity modulated radiation therapy
SRT, SBRT	Stereotactic (body) radiotherapy
EPID	Electronic portal imaging device
MV	Megavolt
kV	Kilovolt
DRR	Digitally reconstructed radiograph
QA	Quality assurance
MVCT, MVCBCT	Megavolt (cone-beam) computed tomography
kVCBCT	Kilovolt cone-beam computed tomography
OBI	On-board imaging system
GTV	Gross tumour volume
CTV	Clinical target volume
PTV	Planning target volume

The Rationale of Image Guidance in Radiation Therapy

Radiation therapy has always been guided by images and many aspects of the treatment process make use of imaging modalities starting at tumour diagnosis and staging of the disease, continuing with treatment simulation and radiation therapy planning, patient positioning (setup), tumour localization and, in a last step, assessment of tumour response to treatment.

CT-based treatment planning and treatment verification make regular use of different types and combinations of imaging. The inclusion of modern imaging modalities incorporating functional or biological information into target delineation has been described in veterinary medicine.[1-3] While the term "image-guided radiotherapy" (IGRT) includes the functional and biological aspect of tumour tissue, the classical, daily use in veterinary medicine focuses on the use of imaging to adjust for positioning errors, adjust for target variations or motion and even, in some cases, adapt treatment to tumour response.

The goal of IGRT is to improve accuracy in radiation therapy and thereby reduce normal tissue toxicity. By improving the accuracy of the radiation field placement, the applied margins for uncertainties can be reduced, resulting in lower side effects or allowing for increased radiation dose to the tumour. The reduction of the planning target volume margins is a very important area of improvement for clinical radiotherapy strategies, such as 3D-conformal radiotherapy, as well as for other techniques, such as intensity modulated radiotherapy (IMRT) and stereotactic (body) radiotherapy (SRT, SBRT).

During a course of treatment, several factors contribute to differences between the planned dose distribution and the effectively delivered dose. One such factor is uncertainty in patient position on the treatment unit. IGRT is a component of the radiation therapy process that incorporates imaging coordinates from the treatment plan in order to ensure the patient is properly aligned in the treatment room.

Historical Image Guidance for Treatment

Anatomical landmarks or skin marks can be helpful for setting up a radiation field for certain areas and techniques; however, these aides are mostly useful for superficial tumour treatment. In the early days of radiation therapy megavoltage portal films were used for position localization. While easy to perform and not requiring expensive technical equipment, portal film imaging is not a real-time verification of treatment setup. The assessment of the landmarks used for deviation is facilitated by the magnification on the images, but the quality of megavoltage portal films is poor and hence a severely limiting factor for interpretation of these marks.[4] The use of electronic portal imaging devices (EPIDs) has developed into a tool for accurate field placement and as a quality assurance for review by radiation oncologists. The digital imaging device offers the additional possibility of manipulation and processing of the image, as well as electronic archiving. The spatial resolution of the images is still somewhat limited due to the high-energy (portal) beam of the (megavolt) therapy machine (MV) as well as due to its large focal spot size.[5]

Current In-room Image Guided Radiation Therapy Imaging Modalities

In-room IGRT modalities are mostly related to daily patient setup and treatment delivery. In the simplest form, the images are acquired prior to treatment and used to correct the patient setup so as to align the target with the planned treatment position. Typically, a couch positional adjustment is used to realign the patient. The interfractional modalities are grouped into 2D radiographic and 3D tomographic imaging.[6]

2D Image Guided Radiation Therapy

Two-dimensional radiographic imaging can be further divided into megavoltage (MV) and kilovoltage (kV) x-ray imaging. In both cases, a flat-panel image detector with a matrix of 256×256 amorphous silicon photodiode solid-state detectors are used.[7] For MV imaging (portal imaging), a small amount of the treatment x-ray beam is used to identify the patient's actual setup and compare it to the planned setup using skeletal anatomy or a surrogate, such as implanted radio-opaque fiducial markers. As the same MV beam is used for verification and treatment, this method of verification provides direct in-field (portal) verification of treatment delivery. In other words, the beam aperture itself, including beam-shaping devices, such as multileaf collimators, can be depicted and compared to the planned position. In order to acquire a MV image, a small proportion of dose (usually around 1-5 cGy) is used. The use of a high-energy x-ray beam produces portal images of lower spatial resolution, lower image contrast, and hence poorer image quality due to the large Compton scatter effect.

Two-dimensional kilovoltage x-ray imaging for IGRT is usually provided by a digital imaging system connected to the gantry of the linear accelerator with robotic arms. This system is mounted on retractable arms and the x-ray source and flat-panel detector are orthogonal to the therapy MV beam. As the system is mounted on the gantry, orthogonal kV images can be performed by a gantry rotation of 90 degrees (FIGURE 1A, B). The orthogonal image pairs are then matched to the reference images that consist of digitally reconstructed radiographs (DRRs) from the planning CT, providing means for highly accurate patient position verification (FIGURE 2A). Additionally, most of these systems also have a fluoroscopic imaging mode, which can be used for organ or fiducial marker motion observation. The advantages of kV imaging for verification lies in the superior quality of the images (near-diagnostic quality) especially for aligning skeletal or implanted radio-opaque landmarks. The low imaging dose is in the range of 0.01 to 0.1 cGy per image, which is an additional advantage compared to the MV images (with imaging doses in the range of 1-3 cGy or higher). Regular quality assurance (QA) processes are required in order to ensure and maintain an isocenter alignment of the gantry-mounted

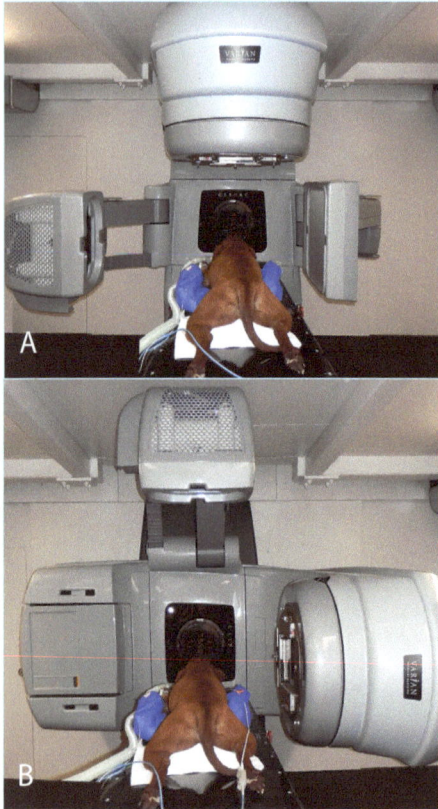

Figure 1. Acquisition of pre-treatment orthogonal kV images: (A) the latero-lateral image allows for correction in the longitudinal and vertical direction, (B) the 180 degree rotated image (dorsoventral) allows for longitudinal, horizontal and rotational correction.

kV imaging beam lines (orthogonal to the treatment beam line) within clinical tolerance.

3D Image Guided Radiation Therapy

Three-dimensional tomographic imaging provides 3D anatomical information and improved soft-tissue visibility, leading to certain advantages over radiographic imaging. Furthermore, the CT images may be used in adaptive radiation therapy, where a treatment plan is modified in response to changes in anatomy. While some older systems combined a linear accelerator and a conventional helical CT unit in the same room, mounting the CT scanner along a pair of rails, the gantry-mounted kV on-board imaging systems (OBI) are capable of cone-beam CT (CBCT). For the CBCT, the two-dimensional area of the detector is used. During the arc rotation of image acquisition, the patient on the treatment table is not moved. The scanned volume along the patient's axis depends on the detector size and is in the range of 15 cm with the full-fan technique. A half-fan technique ("shifted detector") can extend the axial field of view to at least 40 cm, if needed. The reconstruction software allows the conversion into volumetric images using a filtered back-projection algorithm.[7,8]

KVCBCT images are usually acquired with an on-board kV imaging system. The advantage of CBCT for patient position verification is the improved soft-tissue resolution, allowing the depiction of organs at risk within the area of interest. Relative to the below-mentioned MVCBCT images, there is better contrast and spatial resolution with the kV volumetric images, the softtissue visibility is superior at much lower doses to the patient, and the images are compatible with the reference treatment plan images.[6,7] There is 3D/3D matching software which is used to compare the CBCT with the planning CT and sends adjusted position shifts to the treatment table directly (FIGURE 2B). Image contrast is slightly reduced due to high x-ray scatter and kV-CBCT image resolution is

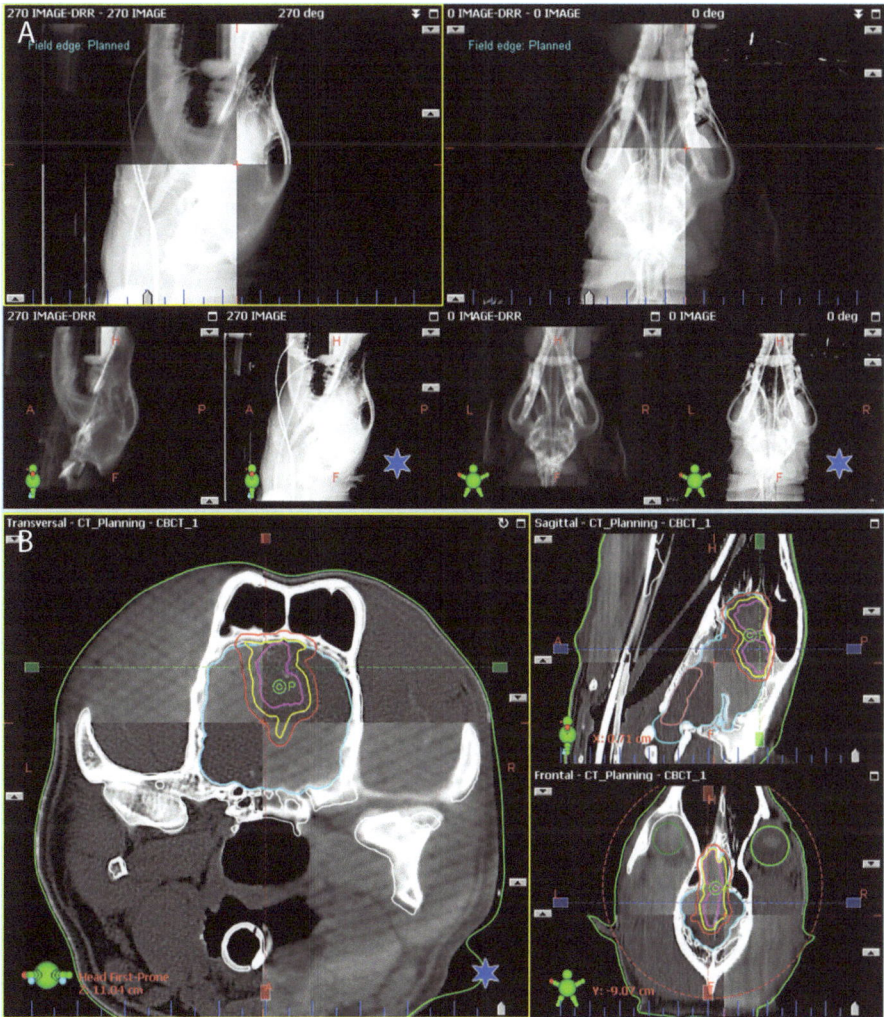

Figure 2. Image registration using the split-window in (A) kV and (B) kVCBCT images. The digitally reconstructed radiographs of the treatment planning CTs (planned position) are overlaid with the verification images of the actual position of the day. Eventual position offset can be directly corrected before treatment.

inferior to diagnostic CT images. Additionally, the speed of gantry rotation is limited, possibly affecting the CBCT image quality due to respiratory motion. Nevertheless the image quality provides an acceptable soft-tissue contrast for target and organ-at-risk localization. For adaptive radiotherapy, CBCTs could also be used for treatment planning. Periodic geometric QA and calibration is needed to maintain image quality and spatial accuracy for CBCT.[6]

Tomotherapy machines (TomoTherapy Inc., Madison, WI) combine helical megavoltage CT (MVCT) with a linear accelerator. Helical tomotherapy treatment uses a continuous gantry and couch motion during treatment, which resembles the motion of a conventional helical CT scanner. With this technology, pretreatment MVCT images can be obtained for the treatment beam line and a field of view of 40 cm can be reconstructed. Due to the energy of the beam for imaging, MVCT image quality is not as high as kVCT, but still provides sufficient contrast for patient position verification.[9] However, an advantage of MVCTs is that the linearity of the MVCT numbers relative to the imaged material electron density corresponds to the physics of the absorbed dose from the therapeutic beam and leads to reliable and accurate dose calculation that can be used in image-guided adaptive radiotherapy. Furthermore, there is less susceptibility to imaging artefacts due to metallic (high atomic number) objects (such as implants). As the traditional EPID with the amorphous silicon flat-panel detector can be used, MVCBCT implementation does not require extensive modification of a linear accelerator.[7,8]

Image Guided Radiation Therapy Requirements

Commissioning and regular QA strategies for all IGRT-imaging system parts are essential and needed to ensure geometric accuracy and optimal image quality. The in-room imaging modality's isocenter needs to be aligned with the treatment radiation isocenter. Mechanical sagging correction is required in order to provide the stringent geometric accuracy for the alignment of the OBI and EPID detectors. The clinically acceptable tolerance must be periodically checked using QA phantoms and is usually referenced to the MV EPID as the gold standard, as the MV EPID provides the treatment beam line reference. The allowed tolerance depends on the treatment techniques used and should be within 2 mm for regular treatment procedures and within 1 mm for stereotactic use.[10]

The alignment of the daily 2D or 3D setup images with the planned reference images (DRR images or planning CT volume) is referred to as image registration. Image registration can be influenced by changes in anatomy, such as daily motion, deformation or physical changes, such as organ filling status and weight gain or loss. Clinically, the focus on registration can be set on anatomical landmarks, such as bones, or directly at the tumour position. In general, verification is performed in two to three orthogonal planar views using tools such as colour blending, split windows or checkerboard. Patient setup corrections can usually be made in three or four degrees of freedom-longitudinal, vertical, horizontal, rotational (yaw)—unless a 6D robotic couch is available (additional pitch and roll correction possible). The final overall setup accuracy for a given tumour localization depends on patient immobilization as well as registration observer variation, registration accuracy, couch adjustment accuracy and imaging-treatment isocenter discrepancy.

Patient Position Correction Strategies

Correction strategies for treatment decisions can be grouped into online approaches, where the adjustment is applied during the current treatment session, or off-line approaches, in which the correction of the patient is determined from previous treatment sessions. The online approach is associated with a higher workload on the treatment machine but results in direct increase in positioning precision. In the anesthetized animal patient, interfractional variations are usually larger than intrafractional ones and therefore pre-treatment setup corrections are usually performed. For large intrafractional motion, such as respiratory motion, real-time monitoring of implanted markers can be used for accurate "gating" of the treatment. Real-time tumour tracking has been implemented for the CyberKnife unit via implanted fiducial markers; however, for regular linear accelerators this capability is still at a developing stage.[11,12]

The institution's patient position, verification and correction strategies must be considered in the determination of planning target volume (PTV)* margins. The chosen PTV margins for the planned area of treatment should ensure minimal geometric systematic and random errors in radiation field placement. With proper patient immobilization techniques, for example, the reported 3-4 mm margin for the treatment of tumours in the head region of dogs can be decreased to 2 mm with in-room image guidance.[13-16] Neglecting to account for daily setup variations will have an adverse effect on clinical outcome, particularly with techniques such as IMRT that yield precise dose distributions tightly conforming to the target with adjacent steep dose gradients. Not only might adjacent normal structures be overdosed, but the target itself may be underdosed, potentially reducing the probability of tumour control.[9,17-22] Hence, the successful implementation of techniques such as IMRT or even SBRT / SRT require daily image guidance to ensure accurate dose delivery. In the case of regions with significant inter- and intrafractional organ variations, such as lung, bladder and prostate tumours, significant changes can occur because of the movement of the surrounding anatomy, such as variable bowel and bladder filling status. Furthermore, target structure variation (tumour shrinkage) is usually not symmetrical but can follow certain trends. For bladder and/or prostate cancers in dogs, a useful technique has been described to adjust the PTV expansion required to account tor the day-to-day movement of bladder and colon.[23-26]

---

* The volumes referred to in radiotherapy are as follows: GTV (gross tumour volume): position and extent of gross tumour, i.e. what can be seen, palpated or imaged. CTV (clinical target volume): This second volume contains the GTV, plus a margin for sub-clinical disease spread, which therefore cannot be fully imaged. It is the most difficult because this volume must be adequately treated to achieve cure. PTV (planning target volume): The third volume includes the former two and is designed to allow for uncertainties in planning or treatment delivery. It is a geometric concept designed to ensure that the radiotherapy dose is actually delivered to the CTV.

Conclusion

The application of IGRT to treatment delivery provides improved geometric and dosimetric accuracy in the treatment of localized tumours. This verification technique reduces margins and hence toxicities to surrounding normal tissues, especially for plans with sharp dose gradients or a moving target. Nevertheless, an institutional protocol for correction strategies accounting for the various uncertainties in the treatment process and the individual technical specifications and limitations of the equipment must be developed in order to make best use of the technologic advantages that are provided with the various levels of IGRT.

References

1.   Ballegeer EA, Forrest LJ, Jeraj R, Mackie TR, Nickles RJ. PET/CT following intensity-modulated radiation therapy for primary lung tumor in a dog. *Vet Radiol Ultrasound*. 2006;**47**:228-233.

2.   Sovik A, Malinen E, Skogmo HK, Bentzen SM, Bruland OS, Olsen DR. Radiotherapy adapted to spatial and temporal variability in tumor hypoxia. *Int J Radiat Oncol Biol Phys*. 2007;**68**:1496-1504.

3.   Sovik A, Rodal J, Skogmo HK, Lervag C, Eilertsen K, Malinen E. Adaptive radiotherapy based on contrast enhanced cone beam CT imaging. *Acta Oncol*. 2010;**49**:972-977.

4.   Bissett R, Leszczynski K, Loose S, Boyko S, Dunscombe P. Quantitative vs. subjective portal verification using digital portal images. *Int J Radiat Oncol Biol Phys*. 1996;**34**:489-495.

5.   Munro P, Bouius DC. X-ray quantum limited portal imaging using amorphous silicon flat-panel arrays. *Med Phys*. 1998;**25**:689-702.

6.   Li G, Mageras GS, Dong L, Mohan R. Image-Guided Radiation Therapy. In: Kahn, F, Gerbi, B.J.(ed): *Treatment planning in radiation oncology*. Philadelphia: Lippincott Williams & Wilkins Kluwer, 2012;229-258.

7.   Kahn F, Gibbons JP. Image-Guided Radiation Therapy. *The physics of radiation therapy*. Philadelphia, PA: Lippincott Williams & Wilkins, 2014;510-523.

8.   Cho PS, Rudd AD, Johnson RH. Cone-beam CT from width-truncated projections. *Comput Med Imaging Graph*. 1996;**20**:49-57.

9.   Forrest LJ, Mackie TR, Ruchala K, Turek M, Kapatoes J, Jaradat H, et al. The utility of megavoltage computed tomography images from a helical tomotherapy system for setup verification purposes. *Int J Radiat Oncol Biol Phys*. 2004;**60**:1639-1644.

10. Klein EE, Hanley J, Bayouth J, Yin FF, Simon W, Dresser S, et al. Task Group 142 report: quality assurance of medical accelerators. *Med Phys.* 2009;**36**:4197-4212.

11. Schweikard A, Shiomi H, Adler J. Respiration tracking in radiosurgery. *Med Phys.* 2004;**31**:2738-2741.

12. Stintzing S, Hoffmann RT, Heinemann V, Kufeld M, Muacevic A. Frameless single-session robotic radiosurgery of liver metastases in colorectal cancer patients. *Eur J Cancer.* 2010;**46**:1026-1032.

13. Harmon J, Van Ufflen D, Larue S. Assessment of a radiotherapy patient cranial immobilization device using daily on-board kilovoltage imaging. *Vet Radiol Ultrasound.* 2009;**50**:230-234.

14. Kent MS, Gordon IK, Benavides I, Primas P, Young J. Assessment of the accuracy and precision of a patient immobilization device for radiation therapy in canine head and neck tumors. *Vet Radiol Ultrasound.* 2009;**50**:550-554.

15. Kubicek LN, Seo S, Chappell RJ, Jeraj R, Forrest LJ. Helical tomotherapy setup variations in canine nasal tumor patients immobilized with a bite block. *Vet Radiol Ultrasound.* 2012;**53**:474-481.

16. Rohrer Bley C, Blattmann H, Roos M, Sumova A, Kaser-Hotz B. Assessment of a radiotherapy patient immobilization device using single plane port radiographs and a remote computed tomography scanner. *Vet Radiol Ultrasound.* 2003;**44**:470-475.

17. Deveau MA, Gutierrez AN, Mackie TR, Tome WA, Forrest LJ. Dosimetric impact of daily setup variations during treatment of canine nasal tumors using intensity-modulated radiation therapy. *Vet Radiol Ultrasound.* 2010;**51**:90-96.

18. Glasser SA, Charney S, Dervisis NG, Witten MR, Ettinger S, Berg J, et al. Use of an image-guided robotic radiosurgery system for the treatment of canine nonlymphomatous nasal tumors. *J Am Anim Hosp Assoc.* 2014;**50**:96-104.

19. Kippenes H, Gavin PR, Parsaei H, Phillips MH, Cho PS, Leathers CW, et al. Spatial accuracy of fractionated IMRT delivery studies in canine paraspinal irradiation. *Vet Radiol Ultrasound.* 2003;**44**:360-366.

20. Kippenes H, Gavin PR, Sande RD, Rogers D, Sweet V. Accuracy of positioning the cervical spine for radiation therapy and the relationship to GTV, CTV and PTV. *Vet Radiol Ultrasound.* 2003;**44**:714-719.

21. Lawrence JA, Forrest LJ, Turek MM, Miller PE, Mackie TR, Jaradat HA, et al. Proof of principle of ocular sparing in dogs with sinonasal tumors treated with intensity-modulated radiation therapy. *Vet Radiol Ultrasound.* 2010;**51**:561-570.

22. Vaudaux C, Schneider U, Kaser-Hotz B. Potential for intensity-modulated radiation therapy to permit dose escalation for canine nasal cancer. *Vet Radiol Ultrasound.* 2007;**48**:475-481.

23. Harmon J, Jr., Yoshikawa H, Custis J, Larue S. Evaluation of canine prostate intrafractional motion using serial cone beam computed tomography imaging. *Vet Radiol Ultrasound.* 2013;**54**:93-98.

24. Nieset JR, Harmon JF, Johnson TE, Larue SM. Comparison of adaptive radiotherapy techniques for external radiation therapy of canine bladder cancer. *Vet Radiol Ultrasound.* 2014;**55**:644-650.

25. Nieset JR, Harmon JF, Larue SM. Use of cone-beam computed tomography to characterize daily urinary bladder variations during fractionated radiotherapy for canine bladder cancer. *Vet Radiol Ultrasound.* 2011;**52**:580-588.

26. Nolan MW, Kogan L, Griffin LR, Custis JT, Harmon JF, Biller BJ, et al. Intensity-modulated and image-guided radiation therapy for treatment of genitourinary carcinomas in dogs. *J Vet Intern Med.* 2012;**26**:987-995.

3   DIAGNOSTIC IMAGING OF THE EQUINE BACK

Fabrice Audigié, Virginie Coudry, Sandrine Jacquet, Lélia Bertoni, Jean-Marie Denoix

École Nationale Vétérinaire d'Alfort, Maisons Alfort, France

Diagnostic Imaging: Progress in the Knowledge of Equine Back Lesions

Back problems are a major cause of poor performance and gait abnormalities in sports and racehorses, but the definitive diagnosis of the cause of back pain remains a complex task for the equine veterinarian. The first step is a detailed clinical examination with the objectives of determining whether back pain is present, documenting the associated functional abnormalities and clinical signs and obtaining a differential diagnosis (neck, back or pelvic injuries). The next step is the identification of the cause of pain using diagnostic imaging techniques. Imaging of the spine is still challenging in horses because the thoracolumbar spine is a large area covered by thick muscles and contains numerous joints of different types—the syndesmosis between the spinous processes (SP) of the vertebrae, the synovial intervertebral articulation (SIVA), the symphysis between the vertebral bodies (VB) and the synovial costovertebral articulations. In the last twenty-five years, marked improvement in the radiographic and ultrasonographic assessment of the thoracolumbar area has been achieved. With appropriate radiographic equipment, back imaging can be performed routinely in the standing horse to achieve a definitive diagnosis of back injuries. This approach can be complemented by nuclear scintigraphy in more complex clinical cases or to go further in the documentation and diagnosis of back conditions. The purpose of this paper is first to describe some technical aspects of equine back imaging and then to present reference images and most frequent conditions encountered in sports and racehorses.

Imaging Modalities: Indications, Technical Aspects and Practical Uses

Indications

There are numerous problems that may indicate diagnostic imaging of the equine back. Complaints by the owner, rider or trainer about the racing and sports uses of horses (particularly for poor performance) is one of the most frequent reasons for performing back imaging. Physical examination can show muscle atrophy in the thoracolumbar area, which is usually diffuse and bilateral. This amyotrophy may also be observed in the caudal cervical and pelvic regions due to the biomechanical interactions between neck, back and pelvic movement. Conversely, focal or diffuse swellings are sometimes found. Back pain and stiffness, defence reactions and abnormal heat are other local symptoms. Dynamic examination is a crucial step that can be performed in hand, on the lunge and ridden. Its advantage is to be less sensitive to individual behavioural reactions compared to physical examination. Reduced back mobility, restricted gait with short strides, especially on short circles, and poor hindlimb propulsion and/or engagement are frequent symptoms associated with back injuries. On the circle, the horse may also have a tendency to lean the body toward the direction of the circle rather than bend the trunk. Finally the examination of the horse performing its discipline (eg. jumping, dressage) or under racing conditions may reveal other disorders compatible with back injuries.

Radiography

Radiographic examination of the back is technically challenging and can be performed routinely in the standing sedated horse if dedicated equipment is available. This modality allows documentation of numerous lesions from the 1st thoracic vertebra (T1) to the 4th lumbar vertebra (L4) in an adult horse. In terms of diagnostic information, this represents the most cost-effective examination. The radiographic technique used has been described previously.[1-3] A powerful X-ray generator of 80 kW, and optimally 100 kW, is necessary for imaging the caudal thoracic and lumbar regions. Due to the thickness of the equine back, a focused grid with a ratio of 10 to 12 limits the scattering and consequently improves the diagnostic quality of the radiographs, particularly for the SIVA. This grid should ideally be placed in a ceiling suspension system. A stand-alone rolling cassette holder may also be used but requires accurate positioning to avoid grid cutoff artifacts. Images are obtained with the horse sedated and standing squarely on its four limbs with the head placed on a dedicated support.[4] Radiographs are acquired at the end of expiration phase in an attempt to limit superimposition of the ribs and diaphragm over the caudal thoracic SIVA. Compared to old conventional radiographic techniques, computed radiographic (CR) and digital systems (DR) permit visualization in

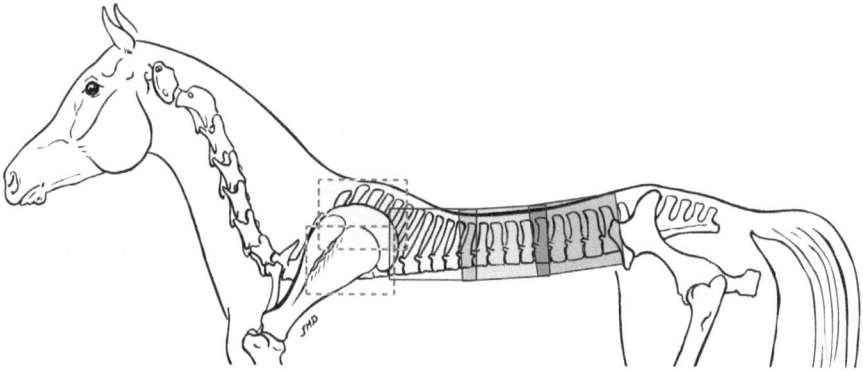

Figure 1. Diagram of lateral radiographic projections of the spine performed with CR and DR systems. Three global images (grey squares - solid line border) are acquired: mid thoracic, caudal thoracic and lumbar regions. Two projections (caudal thoracic and lumbar areas) focused on the SIVA and VB or 1 centered on the thoracolumbar junction may be added particularly in large horses for obtaining higher quality images (not shown). When indicated, an additional view of the withers (grey square - dashed line) and one of the cranial thoracic spine (white square - dashed line) are also acquired.

the same image of the entire vertebrae from the dorsal most extent of the SP to the ventral part of the vertebral bodies. Such an image requires the use of an aluminium wedge filter placed on the back of the horse to compensate for the large differences in thickness of the body parts radiographed. Finally, a moving grid (Potter-Bucky) or post-processing algorithms with a stationary grid should be used with CR and DR systems to avoid Moiré artifacts (optical interference between grid lines and image pixels) on the radiographic images.

Four to five lateral exposures are routinely obtained using large flat panel detectors or cassettes for a detailed and complete evaluation of the thoracolumbar spine between the 8th thoracic vertebra (T8) and 4th lumbar vertebra (L4). Two additional lateral views can be added if disorders of the withers or cranial thoracic spine are suspected (Figure 1). Moreover, lateral 20° dorsal oblique projections for the thoracic SIVA can also be performed to separately evaluate the left and right joints.[5]

Exposure factors depend on the radiographic equipment used. Table 1 presents examples of exposure factors used with a CR system. CR radiographic images of SIVA and VB for the caudal part of the back are frequently underexposed for large horses (600 kg and more) even with such exposure factors. Higher quality radiographs of the back are obtained with DR systems compared to CR ones, particularly in these large horses, due to the higher detective quantum efficiency (DQE) and greater dynamic range of DR technologies.

Radiographic image	kV	mAs
Global image		
Mid thoracic area (T8-T14)	85-90	80-90
Caudal thoracic area (T13-T18)	90-95	125-160
Lumbar area (T18-L4)	105-110	125-160
Focused image SIVA +VB		
(T14-L1)	95-100	125-160
(T18-L4)	110-115	125-180
Additional radiographs		
Withers (T4-T10)	75-80	80-125
Cranial thoracic area SIVA + VB (T1-T8)	110-115	125-180

Table 1. Examples of exposure factors used with a CR system for lateral projections of the spine (Horse: 500-600 kg. Grid: focused, ratio = 12 and focal distance = 115 cm).

Ultrasonography

With progressive improvement of ultrasound equipment, diagnostic quality images of the back can now be obtained routinely. Ultrasound examination of the supraspinous ligament can be performed with 7.5-10 MHz linear or convex transducers.[6] Imaging of the SIVA, transverse processes, dorsal aspects of the ribs and back muscles is best performed with 3 to 6 MHz convex probes. Transverse images made on each side of the vertebral column are more informative when looking for SIVA injuries compared to longitudinal ones because immediate comparison between the left and right side is possible. The objective of this approach is to evaluate the caudal and cranial articular processes as well as the joint space of each intervertebral joint on both sides.

Images are usually acquired over the areas presenting with clinical manifestations (pain and/or restricted mobility) or abnormal radiographic or scintigraphic findings and more systematically for the caudal lumbar region that is not visible radiographically in adult horses.

Finally, ultrasound examination is also performed using a transrectal approach to evaluate the last lumbar VB (L4-L6) and associated intervertebral disks (L4 and L5). The lumbosacral junction is also imaged including the lumbosacral intervetebral disc (L6), the lumbosacral intertransverse joints, the ventral intervertebral foramina, the ventral ramus of the L5 and L6 segmental nerves and the major and minor psoas muscles.[7] This part of back diagnostic imaging will not be described in detail because this examination is mainly conducted during the transrectal ultrasound evaluation of the pelvis.

Nuclear Scintigraphy

The authors recommend that horses are warmed-up whenever possible (i.e., worked on the lunge, ridden or on a track) for 15-20 minutes before radiopharmaceutical injection of 1 GBq per 100 kg of 99mTechnetium-dicarboxypropane diphosphonate (99mTc-DPD, CisBio International, France). Bone phase images are acquired 3 hours later using a rectangular gamma-camera equipped with a low energy, high resolution collimator. Each static image of 1-minute duration and 128×128 matrix size is calculated using a homemade motion correction software applied to the corresponding dynamic acquisition of 30 images of 2 seconds duration.

The thoracolumbar spine is routinely examined with two lateral oblique views on both sides including a dorsolateral view of the thoracic spine (approximately from T5 to T17, depending on the size of the horse) and a dorsolateral view of the lumbar spine (approximately from T15 to the iliac crest). In these views, the camera is angled approximately 45° ventral from vertical to place the camera as close as possible to the SP, SIVA and VB compared to smaller angles used by other authors. For example, Gillen et al. 2009 acquired images with an angle of 20° ventral from vertical and Erichsen et al. 2004 with an angle of 30°. The advantages of these lower angle projections is to provide a closer image to the radiographic one and to minimize superimposition of the SP and SIVA with potential radiation coming from the kidneys, particularly the right one. In contrast, the signal to noise ratio of the spine is lower compared to the more oblique projections because gamma rays must go through larger muscle volume.

These four back views are completed by one horizontal dorsal image performed over the lumbo-sacro-iliac junction including also most of the lumbar region. This projection is particularly useful for detecting transitional vertebrae at the lumbosacral junction and malalignment of lumbar SP associated with overriding SP. This last view can also be obtained for the thoracic and withers areas, but this is not performed routinely in our whole body examination due to their lower diagnostic performance.

Imaging Uses

Diagnostic Procedures

Horses presenting with clinical signs of back disorders routinely undergo the following examinations:

- Radiographic examination of the back (T8-L4: 4 to 5 lateral radiographic projections) and one lateral radiograph of the caudal cervical region (C5-T1: frequently associated to the corresponding ultrasound examination) because caudal cervical spine injuries may induce clinical signs mimicking back pain.

- Ultrasound evaluation of the lumbar area (T18-L6) with a special interest in its caudal part (L4-L6) not imaged by radiographs and also the abnormal radiographic SIVA.

- Transrectal ultrasound examination of the caudal lumbar area (L4-L6) and of the other pelvic structures, again because of the possible association between clinical signs induced by back and pelvic injuries.

In the same way, routine views of the pelvic and caudal cervical regions are performed in horses referred for scintigraphic examination of the back.

Therapeutic Procedures: Ultrasound Guided Injections

One major interest of diagnostic imaging in back conditions is to precisely define the location of the injured sites, particularly for SIVA injuries. Knowing this, therapeutic deep paramedian ultrasound guided injections (USGI) of the abnormal SIVA can be performed with excellent reliability. With such an approach,[7,8] the therapeutic agent can be injected below the fascia separating the longissimus muscle from the multifidus one, almost in contact with the SIVA or in some cases even within the SIVA itself.

Reference Images and Pathological Findings

Spinous Processes and Associated Ligaments

Kissing spines are the most frequent injuries, but lesions can also affect the supraspinous ligament.

Supraspinous Ligament

The normal supraspinous ligament (SSL) is thicker in the lumbar spine than in the thoracic spine. On transverse sections it is located between the thick and echogenic left and right thoracolumbar fascia. On longitudinal sections the linear achitectural pattern of the ligament can be assessed (Figure 2). As the deep fasciculi are oriented obliquely and ventrocaudally to insert on the following spinous process, they are not perpendicular to the insonating ultrasound beam and thus appear less echogenic than superficial fasciculi on median longitudinal sections. In the withers, the SSL is wide and thin and is in contact with the irregular apophyseal centers of ossification of the cranial thoracic spinous processes.

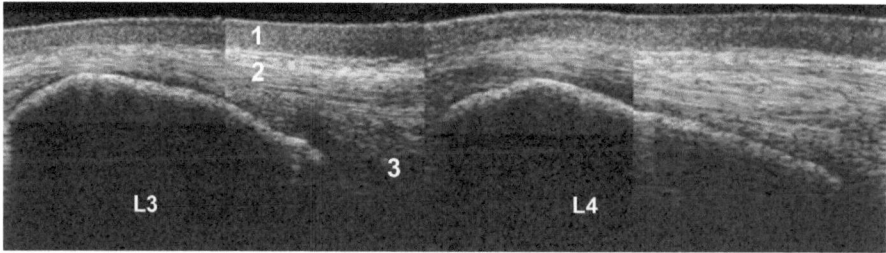

Figure 2. Reference longitudinal ultrasonographic images of the normal supraspinous ligament (SSL) at the level of the L3-L4 vertebrae. The regular longitudinal fascicular architecture of the ligament is clearly visible. Skin and subcutaneous tissue (1), SSL (2), interspinous ligament (3).

SSL injuries (FIGURE 3) are most frequently observed between T14 and L3-6,[9-11] and may induce local deformation (elevation of the dorsal profile or transverse thickening) or pain particularly in acute stages. Recently, no differences in the occurrence of SSL injuries in the thoracic area were found between ridden horses, unridden horses and horses with back pain.[9]

With low exposure radiographs, soft tissue thickening and some focal increased radiopacities may be seen in chronic cases.[10] This increased radiopacity should be differentiated from periligamentous or subcutaneous back mineralisations such as those found in some granulomas. Avulsion fractures or bone remodeling and sclerosis of the dorsal surface of the spinal processes may also be noted.[10]

Abnormal ultrasound findings of the SSL are similar to any desmopathy or entheseopathy and include thickening, changes in echogenicity, alterations of the architectural fiber pattern and/or abnormal bone surface of the tips of the spinous processes. The sensitivity and specificity of the ultrasonographic evaluation of the supraspinous ligament increases when the suspected area is compared with the adjacent cranial and caudal ones using the same transducer positioning.

Acute or subacute desmopathies can cause dorsoventral or transverse thickening of the ligament and reduced echogenicity and may create severe alterations of the linear fiber pattern. They can be found in the median plane or may be asymmetrical. In old or chronic injuries, the ligament often remains thicker with reduced echogenicity and an irregular architectural pattern. Hyperechoic images with or without acoustic shadows are compatible with mineralisation or calcification of the SSL. Alteration of the bone surface of the top of the spinous processes is indicative of enthesopathy of the SSL. When a deformation of the dorsal midline of the back is present, the differential diagnosis between SSL injuries and other periligamentous or subcutaneous injuries can be done with ultrasonography.

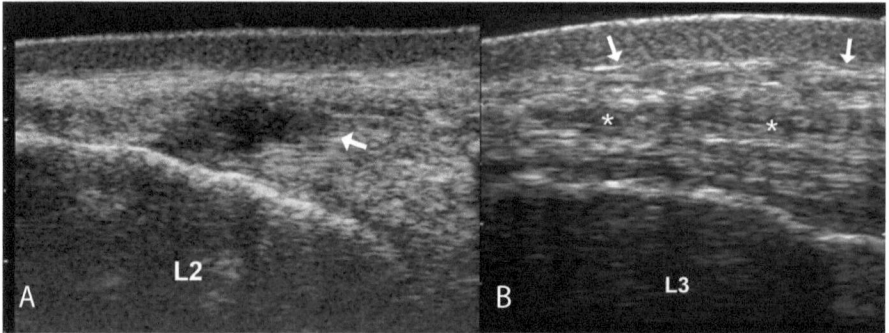

Figure 3. Sagittal ultrasound images of acute and chronic injury of the supraspinous ligament (SSL) in a horse. A: Recent injury of the SSL in an international showjumper. A focal, strongly hypoechoic lesion (arrow) is visible close to the SSL enthesis on the top of L2 with severe fiber pattern alteration (loss of fibers in the center of the lesion). B: Chronic injury of the SSL over the L3 SP with enlargement (note the convex shape of the skin profile) and patchy heterogenous echogenicity (arrows) with more severe hypoechoic areas (*). The irregular aspect of the dorsal bone surface of L2 SP is due to bone remodeling at the enthesis of the SSL.

Spinous Processes

The most frequent injury of the spinous processes (SP) is represented by "kissing spines".[11-16] Kissing spines include different types of injuries including narrowing of the interspinous space, impinging and overriding spinous processes and enthesopathies or desmopathies of the interspinous ligaments. They are most frequently observed in the mid and caudal thoracic area, between T10 and T18. Kissing spines can also been seen in the lumbar area and are even frequently observed without any associated clinical signs between L4 and L5 due to the changes of orientation of the most caudal lumbar spinous processes.

Radiographic examination represents the most cost-effective examination for identification and documentation of kissing spines. SP injuries have been graded radiographically on a 4-grade scale[12] and more recently using a more detailed 7-grade scale.[15] In both scales, severity of the lesions increases from narrowing of the interspinous space to impinging and overriding spinous processes. The degree of bone remodelling, particularly the number of radiolucencies induced by bone lysis, worsens the grade of the lesions (FIGURE 4). More recently, the effect of head and neck position on radiographic measurements of intervertebral distances between thoracic dorsal spinous processes in clinically sound horses has been quantified.[4] Results of this study show that a low head and neck position increased intervertebral distances between adjacent thoracic dorsal spinous processes from the 8th to 15th dorsal spinous processes whereas a high head and neck position had the opposite effect.

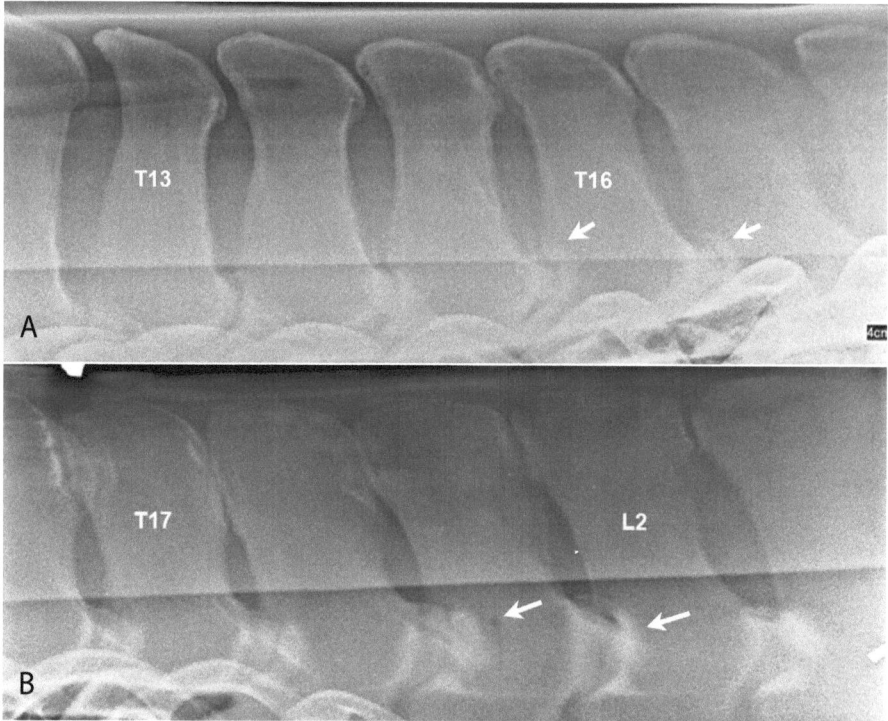

Figure 4. A: Lateral radiographic image of the thoracic SP and corresponding SIVA in an 8-year-old Selle Français showjumper presenting defense reactions when worked. Grade 1 (narrowing of the interspinous space with mild sclerosis of the cortical margins of the SP: T13-T14, T14-T15 and T16-T17) and grade 2 (loss of the interspinous space with moderate sclerosis of the cortical margins of the SP: T15-T16) kissing spines are visible between T13 and T17. Note also the presence of type 4 SIVA arthropathies between T15-T16 and T16-T17 (arrows), other SIVA appear radiographically normal. B: Lateral radiographic image of the thoracolumbar SP and corresponding SIVA in a 3-year-old Thoroughbred flat racing horse presenting with clinical signs of back pain. Grades 2 (L1-L2 and L2-L3) and 3 (severe sclerosis of the cortical margins of the SP or radiuolucent areas: T16-T17, T17-T18 and to a lower degree T18-L1) kissing spines are visible between T16 and L3. Note also the presence of SIVA arthropathies from T17 to L3, more severe between T18 and L2 (arrows: types 2 and 4).

Abnormal findings can also be seen in the ventral part of the spinous processes with irregular bony proliferations of the cranial and/or caudal borders of the SP. These interspinous enthesopathies are frequently not clinically significant when observed alone, for instance in the withers and cranial and mid thoracic spine. In contrast, their clinical significance seems higher if they affect the ventral aspect of the SP and are associated with osteoarthrosis of the articular processes (most frequently type 4 SIVA injuries). Similarly, the severity of the SP lesions was significantly associated with the presence of SIVA osteoarthritis.[15]

Ultrasound examination is of more limited interest for documentation of kissing spines. It can be used to demonstrate contact and/or remodeling between two adjacent spinal processes as well as abnormal alignement between them. Ultrasound is also useful to assess concomittant supraspinous ligament injuries. In most patients, bone scintigraphic images have a high correlation with radiographic ones, both in terms of location and grade of the SP lesions.[12,15] Nuclear scintigraphy is a useful technique to demonstrate the craniocaudal extension of bone remodeling associated with kissing lesions as well as the dorsoventral extension of them. In our experience, grade 3 to 4 lesions of the dorsal part of the spinous processes are often, if not always, associated with increased radiopharmaceutical uptake (IRU), confirming the potential clinical incidence of these lesions (FIGURE 5). However, it's important to remember that IRU is not synonymous with pain, and horses with SIVA osteoarthrosis are more likely to have thoracolumbar pain than horses with lesions of the SPs alone.[12,16]

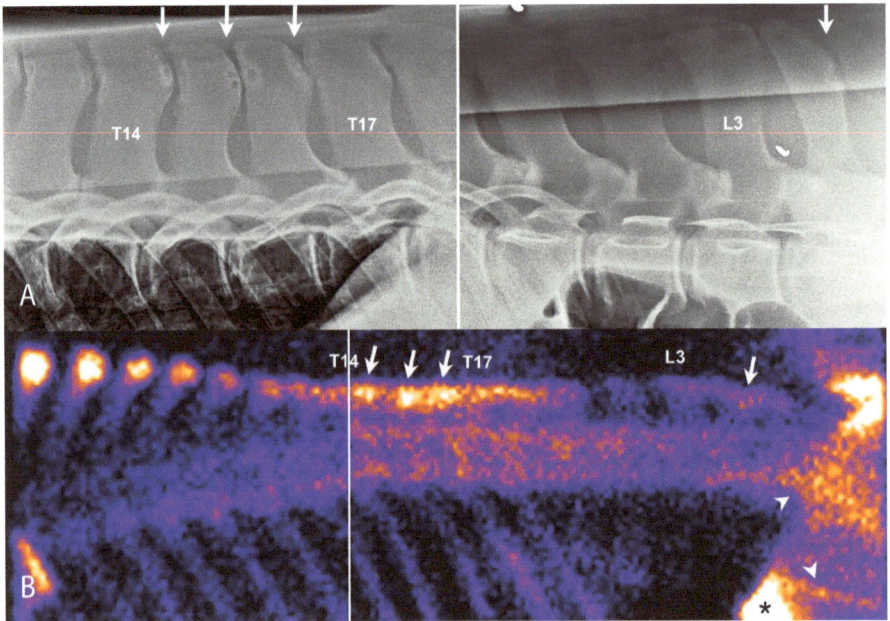

Figure 5. Reconstructed lateral radiographic image of the thoracolumbar spine (A) and corresponding reconstructed oblique left thoracolumbar scintigraphic image (B) in a 2-year-old Thoroughbred flat racing horse presenting with clinical signs of back pain and left hindlimb lameness. There is strong correlation between the severity of the kissing spines between T14 and T17 (grades 3 [T14-T15, T16-T17] and 4: severe sclerosis of the cortical margins of the SP, osteolysis and change in shape of the SP: T15-T16) and the corresponding IRU (arrows). Other kissing spines (grade 3: T12-T13, T13-T14; grade 2: T17-T18, T18-L1 and grade 1: L3-L4) are less active on the scintigraphic image. Note also the kissing spines between L3-L5 (grade 2) with a mild IRU between L4-L5 (arrow). There is also an IRU in the left gluteal muscles (arrowheads) over the corresponding iliac wing. The left tuber coxae is indicated (*).

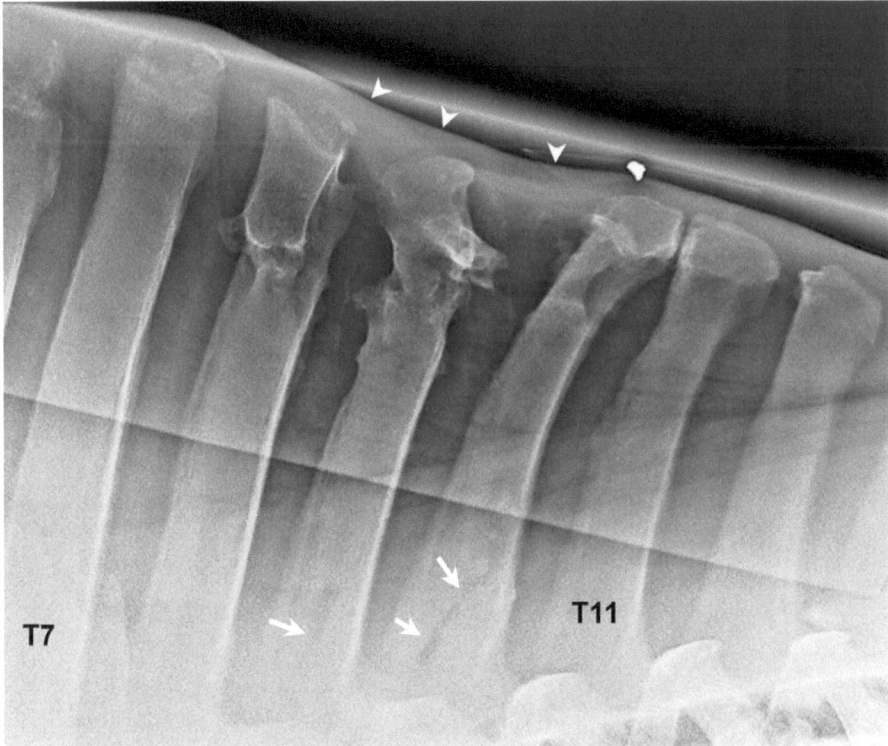

Figure 6. Lateral radiographic image of the withers in a 14-year-old amateur showjumper presented for neck stiffness. An abnormal concave aspect of the dorsal midline skin profile was identified during the physical examination (arrowheads) without any known previous traumatic event. Old fractures and severe remodeling of the proximal part of T8, T9 and T10 SP were found. An oblique radiolucent line with smooth margins (arrows) was also visible at the base of the T9 and T10 SP. These alterations are strongly suggestive of old healed fractures at the base of these SP and also explain the abnormal orientation of T10 SP. There also appears to be some mineralisation of the interspinous ligament associated with the fractured SP.

The frequency and clinical incidence of kissing spines seem to vary according to the horse's discipline and biomechanical solicitations of the equine back in specific gaits and types of exercise and age (extent and grade being more severe in older horses). Generally speaking, these lesions are commonly found in racing thoroughbreds and seem to be tolerated in many of them. They are quite rare in French trotters, but when present, their incidence of clinical signs seems higher. Intermediate frequency and incidence are observed in sport horses. Kissing spines can be found in performing race and sport horses without back pain and even those with normal thoracolumbar mobilisation tests.[13] Thus a careful assessment of the clinical significance of these lesions must be performed on each clinical case.

Fractures of the SP are most frequently seen in the withers region following a traumatic event. Clinical findings of these horses are strongly suggestive with abnormal shape of the dorsal midline of the withers or "sunk" or "flat" withers. In acute stages, swelling, local pain and back stiffness are frequently observed. Radiographic examination determines the number of fractured SP, the proximo-distal location of the fractures, the associated displacement and the presence of bony fragments (FIGURE 6). Despite the dramatic appearance of this injury, the prognosis can remain favourable with conservative treatment and adequate management, such as the use of a purpose-fitted saddle.[17]

SIVA Injuries

The thoracolumbar SIVA are composed of the caudal articular processes (AP) of one vertebra, the cranial AP of the following vertebra and other synovial joint structures (articular cartilage, synovial fluid and membrane, articular capsule). In horses, SIVA are frequently affected with osteoarthrosis, and diagnostic imaging of this condition is crucial in the evaluation of back pain and associated poor performance.

Radiographic Examination

The appearance of normal SIVA on lateral radiographic projections changes along the thoracolumbar spine (FIGURE 7).[1,18] The radiolucent cartilaginous joint space is thin and more clearly defined in the thoracic region, where the articular facets are flat in the lumbar area because of the condylar shape of the AP. Between the mid- and caudal thoracic regions (T12-T16), the radiolucent joint space presents a V shape with a cranial branch oblique dorsocaudally and a shorter caudal branch vertically orientated. At the thoracolumbar junction (T17-T18), the joint space is more difficult to distinguish. In the lumbar region, only the part of the articular surface tangential to the X-ray beam is visible as a linear radiolucent line, obliqued approximately 45° dorsocaudally. The subchondral bone of the cranial AP describes a triangular or V-shaped opacity with the tip of the V being orientated cranially just below this line. Dorsal to this radiolucent joint space, the caudal AP also forms a regular, homogeneous bone opacity. Finally, mamillary processes originating from the cranial AP are superimposed on the SIVA. These mamillary processes extend further dorsally in the thoracic area than in the lumbar one.

SIVA injuries have been classified radiographically into 8 types (TABLE 2 AND FIGURE 8). These abnormal findings are mainly observed at the thoracolumbar junction and in the lumbar area (T15-L4), with a preferential location in the lumbar region for types 5, 7 and 8. In horses presenting for back pain and/or poor performance, there were commonly 2 to 5 affected SIVA per horse, and sclerosis, periarticular bone remodelling and narrowing of the joint space were the most frequent radiographic lesion type.[19]

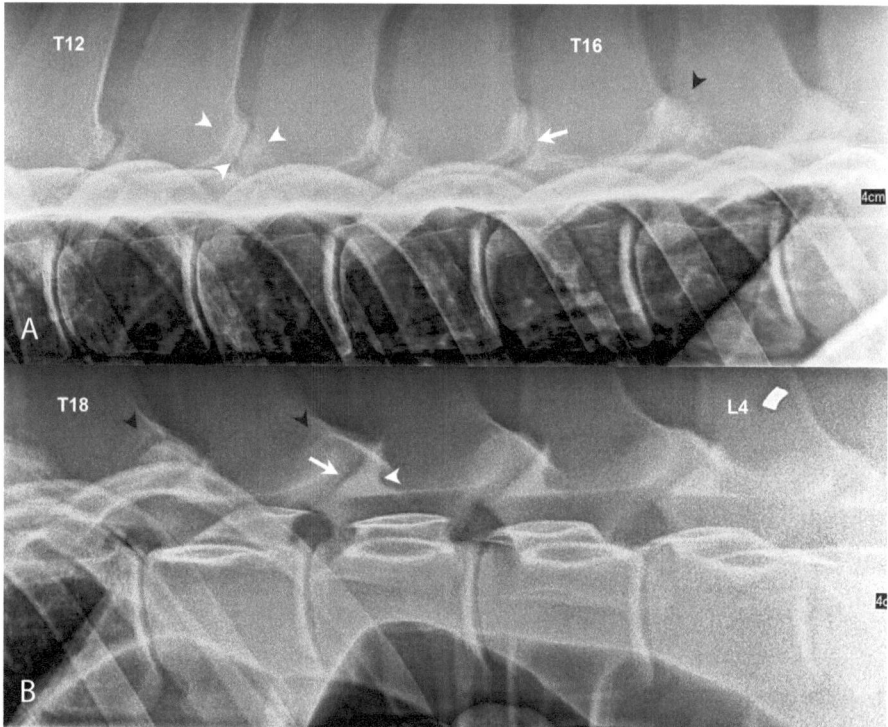

Figure 7. Appearance of normal thoracic and lumbar SIVA on lateral radiographic projections. A: Lateral radiographic image of mid and caudal thoracic SIVA in an 8-year-old intermediate-level Selle-Français show jumper. The radiolucent joint space presents a V shape between T12-T16, with a cranial branch oblique dorsocaudally and a shorter caudal branch vertically orientated (arrow). At the thoracolumbar junction (T17-T18), the joint space is more difficult to distinguish. The mamillary processes are well visible in the thoracic area (white arrowheads). Note the mild periarticular remodeling in T17-T18 SIVA (black arrowhead). B: Lateral radiographic image of the lumbar SIVA in a 5-year-old racing Trotteur. In this lumbar region, the articular surface tangential to the X-ray beam is visible as a linear radiolucent line, obliqued approximately 45° dorsocaudally (arrow). The subchondral bone of the cranial AP describes a triangular or V-shaped opacity, with the tip of the V being orientated cranially (white arrowhead) just below this line. Note the mild periarticular remodeling in T18-L1 and L1-L2 SIVA (black arrowhead).

All abnormal radiographic features described in Table 2 were found in middle-aged and older horses as well as in young racehorses and sport horses from 3 to 6 years old. Changes of these injuries over time is usually slow.

In our experience, SIVA lesions are much more likely associated with back pain than kissing spines or any other vertebral injury. Horses with impingement of the dorsal spinous processes and osteoarthritis had more clinical signs and were generally clinically worse than horses with SP injuries alone.[19] In our experience and as discussed for the kissing spines, the frequency and clinical incidence of SIVA lesions seem to vary according to the horse's discipline. These

Type	Lesion	Abnormal radiographic finding
1	Asymmetry	No clear joint space, double joint space
2	Modification of opacity of the AP	Sclerosis of the subchondral bone Increased opacity of the SIVA
3		Radiolucent areas in the subchondral bone Increased opacity of the AP
4	Periarticular proliferation	Dorsal periarticular proliferation Increased size of the SIVA Often associated opacity alterations of the subchondral bone
5		Ventral periarticular proliferation
6	Ankylosis	Dorsal bridge between 2 following vertebrae
7		Osteolysis of the SIVA, no visble joint space
8	Fracture	Radiolucent line on the caudal or cranial AP

Table 2. Classification of radiographic abnormalities of SIVA injuries.[12,18]

lesions are commonly found in racing thoroughbreds and seem compatible with racing activities in most individuals. They are quite rare in French trotters, but when present, their clinical significance seems higher. Sport horses are intermediate in terms of frequency and severity of injuries. The clinical significance of similar radiographic findings may change greatly depending on individual parameters but also on the influence of the rider and/or exercise types and programs.

Ultrasonographic Examination

Comparative left and right transverse images performed at the same intervetebral level are particularly useful for detecting SIVA lesions. On normal SIVA, left and right joints should be symmetrical, and the dorsal profile of the APs is imaged as a regular, smooth bony contour. From medial-to-lateral the following structures are found:

- The caudal AP of the cranial vertebra in continuity with the adjacent spinous process or interspinous ligament

- The dorsal limit of the synovial joint space, with a small anechoic notch representing the joint space itself separating two smooth articular margins

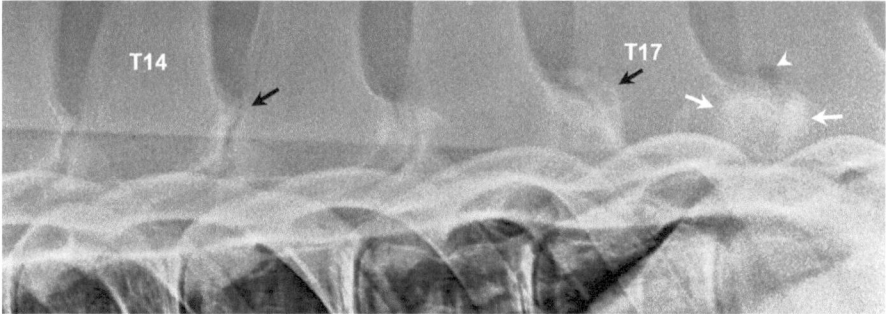

Figure 8. Lateral radiographic image of caudal thoracic SIVA in a 3-year-old high-level Thoroughbred race horse with excellent performances despite a back sensitivity. Severe T16-T17 and T17-T18 SIVA lesions are visible with marked sclerosis (Type 2, white arrows), focal osteolysis (Type 3, arrowhead) and dorsal proliferations (Type 4, black arrows). A lower grade lesion is also found on T14-T15 with dorsal proliferations associated with an abnormal shape of the most dorsal aspect of the articular space.

- The cranial AP of the caudal vertebra bordered laterally by the mamillary process. This process is high in the caudal thoracic region and separated from the AP but is lower and closer to the AP in the lumbar area

- The SIVA are covered by the multifidus muscle, separated from the thick longissimus muscle by an echogenic fascia.

Abnormal findings include left to right asymmetry of the SIVA, loss of joint space identification due to periarticular osteophytes, and dorsal periarticular proliferations (types 4 and 6). Ultrasound is particularly useful to determine whether the proliferation is symmetrical and, if not, which side is the most severely affected (FIGURE 9).

Scintigraphic Examination

On dorso-lateral bone acquisitions, the normal SIVA appear slightly more active than the spinous processes and the vertebral body axis. They present a relatively homogeneous uptake from the cranial thoracic area to the lumbosacral joint with an increased signal in the thoracolumbar junction area (T16-L2).

Abnormal SIVA can demonstrate increased radiopharmaceutical uptake in a single SIVA or on several joints. In some cases, IRU can be detected before occurrence of significant radiographic abnormalities. In other cases, because of the attenuation in the thick erector spinae muscle and the frequent chronicity of osteoarthrosis of the SIVA, nuclear scintigraphy is not completely sensitive to detect changes in these structures. In horses with back pain, 26% of SIVA with osteoarthrosis radiographic signs had a normal scintigraphic uptake,

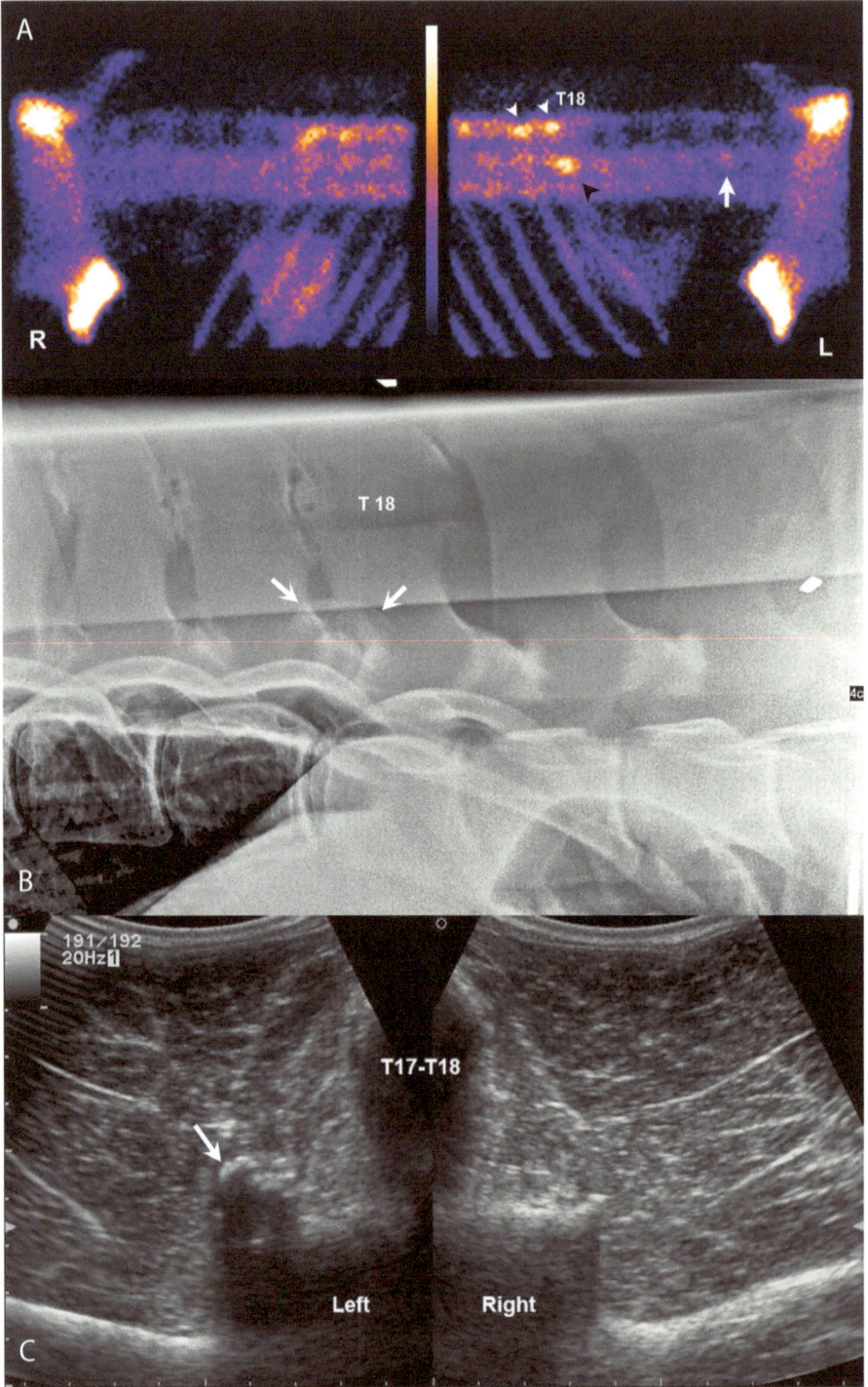

Figure 9. [Opposite page] Correlations between scintigraphic (A: Left image = right oblique dorso-lateral image of the thoracolumbar area; right image = left corresponding image), radiographic (B) and ultrasonographic (C: T17-T18 SIVA) findings in a poorly performing 3-year-old Thoroughbred flat racing horse. This horse presented with clinical signs of back pain, lack of hind-limb propulsion with stiff gaits and galloped frequently with the head in a low position. Marked IRU in the caudal thoracic SP (from T14 to T18 with more severe increased uptakes in T16-T17 and T17-T18: white arrowheads) and in the left T17-T18 SIVA (black arrowhead) are observed on the scintigraphic images (A). A mild IRU is also present in the left L3-L4 SIVA (arrow). Note that this horse has only 5 lumbar vertebrae. The radiographic projection confirms severe kissing spines in the caudal thoracic region (grade 3: T15-T16; grade 4: T16-T17 and T17-T18) and marked osteoarthrosis of T17-18 SIVA (Type 6 = dorsal bridge: arrows). L3-L4 was not visible on this horse due to the superimposition with the iliac wings. Left and right transverse ultrasound (C) images confirm the severe left T17-T18 SIVA lesion (arrow) with periarticular remodeling and dorsal hypertrophy induced by the dorsal bridge. In contrast, a poor correlation is seen between the marked T16-T17 (Type 4) and moderate L1-L2 (Type 2) radiographic SIVA lesions with the corresponding scintigraphic uptakes.

and the strongest association between radiographic abnormalities and scintigraphic ones was seen in horses with intense IRU (Figure 9).[20] For this reason, routine radiographic examination of the back is always performed after scintigraphy for horses presenting with clinical signs of back disorders in our centre. Twenty-six percent of sound horses have mild IRU in the SIVA; however, moderate and severe IRU are more frequently found in horses with back pain (62% of patients).[20]

Other Lesions

Vertebral Body and Intervertebral Disc

With the exception of the caudal lumbar region (L4-S1) evaluated using transrectal ultrasound examination, vertebral bodies and associated intervertebral discs (IVD) are evaluated using radiography. This assessment is facilitated by superimposition of the lungs in the thoracic area. It is more difficult in the lumbar area and the throcolumbar junction because of the presence of the psoas muscles, diaphragm and liver.

Lesions of the vertebral bodies are not commonly found in horses.[11,12,21-23] Vertebral body and IVD abnormalities are observed in thoracolumbar congenital malformations that usually do not induce neurological manifestation. They include mainly transitional abnormalities and vertebral axis deviations such as those observed in foals presenting with thoracolumbar kyphoscoliosis which includes lateral and sagittal deviations as well as rotation of the vertebrae.

Vertebral body fractures have been seen in horses having undergone severe trauma or falls. They can be associated with fractures of the vertebral arches

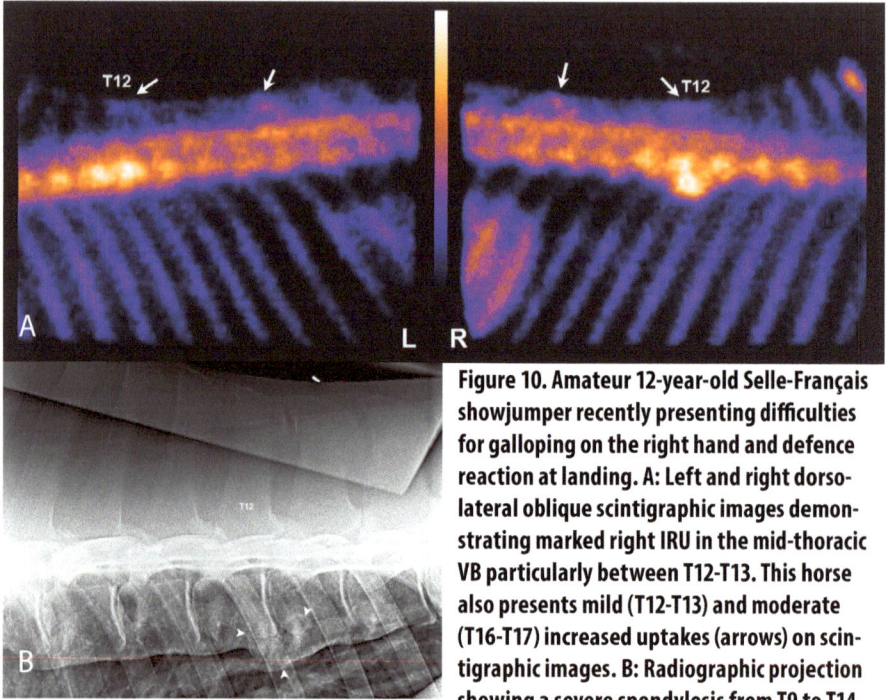

Figure 10. Amateur 12-year-old Selle-Français showjumper recently presenting difficulties for galloping on the right hand and defence reaction at landing. A: Left and right dorso-lateral oblique scintigraphic images demonstrating marked right IRU in the mid-thoracic VB particularly between T12-T13. This horse also presents mild (T12-T13) and moderate (T16-T17) increased uptakes (arrows) on scintigraphic images. B: Radiographic projection showing a severe spondylosis from T9 to T14 with an enlargement and more heteregenous opacity between T12-T13 (arrows). There is also moderate kissing spines between T12-T13 (grade 2 to 3).

and may also be responsible for spinal cord compression inducing hindlimb ataxia and paresis. Recently Collar et al. 2014 have described caudal lumbar vertebral fractures in Quarter and Thoroughbred horses involving the 5th and/or 6th lumbar VB. Vertebral body osteomyelitis inducing neurological manifestations can be seen in the thoracolumbar spine in foals and are frequently associated with spondylodiscitis.[21] Nuclear scintigraphy can be useful to detect severe vertebral body lesions such as fractures and osteomyelitis particularly in the early stages when radiographic alterations are not yet present.

Spondylosis can be detected using radiography and scintigraphy (FIGURE 10), but its prevalence remains low in horses with back pain. Only 3.5% of horses with back pain had radiographic evidence of spondylosis.[23] When complete intervertebral ankylosis is present, there is often more IRU at the cranial and caudal extremities of the affected vertebral segment. Spondylosis may be responsible for back and/or neck pain and/or stiffness in sport and racehorses. It may also represent an incidental finding in low-level performance horses with no history or signs of back pain.

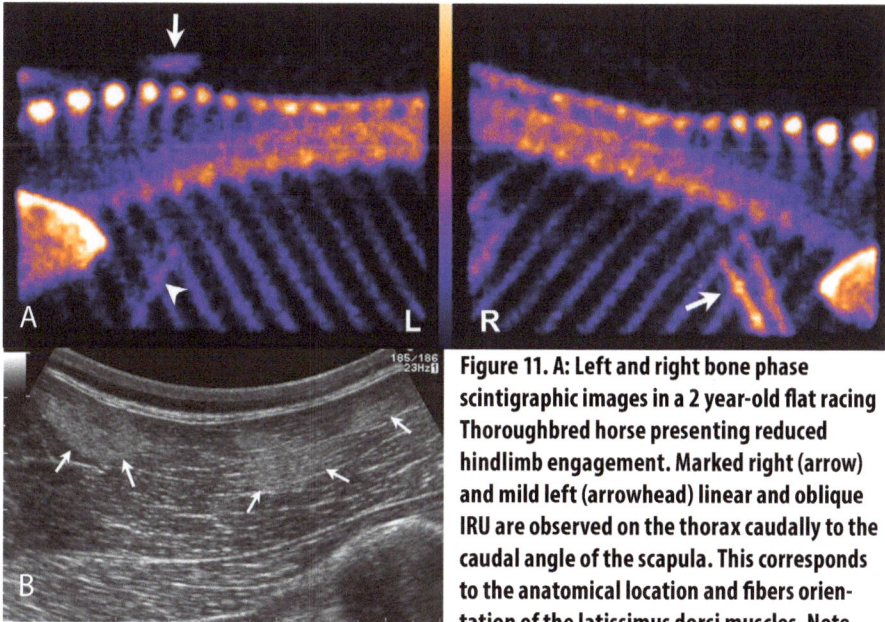

Figure 11. A: Left and right bone phase scintigraphic images in a 2 year-old flat racing Thoroughbred horse presenting reduced hindlimb engagement. Marked right (arrow) and mild left (arrowhead) linear and oblique IRU are observed on the thorax caudally to the caudal angle of the scapula. This corresponds to the anatomical location and fibers orientation of the latissimus dorsi muscles. Note on the left oblique dorsolateral scintigraphic view the rounded IRU of the right latissimus dorsi muscle (arrow) created by the tangential projection with respect to this muscle. B: Transverse ultrasound image of the right latissimus dorsi muscle showing the corresponding typical marble or patchy appearance of the injured muscle with multifocal well-delineated abnormal areas of increased echogenicity.

Ribs and Transverse Processes

On normal images, the dorsal surface of the ribs is convex and the dorsal surface of the transverse process is flat. Thoracolumbar transitional vertebrae are frequently seen with a rib on one side and a transverse process on the opposite side. Abnormal findings and lesions include fractures and lumbar kissing processes. Fractures of one or several ribs can be detected using radiography, ultrasound or scintigraphy, with or without a history of trauma. In the acute and subacute stages, they are associated with back pain and stiffness. Horses may react aggressively if pressure is applied on the affected region.

Back Muscles

Ultrasound is the imaging modality of choice for investigating muscle status and injuries. Nevertheless, bone phase scintigraphic images have also demonstrated a high sensitivity for detecting focal or diffuse exertional myopathies on the pelvic and back muscles with or without significant changes in blood levels of muscle enzymes.[24,25] Muscle injuries appeared most frequently as focal or diffuse linear IRU with specific orientations corresponding to the anatomy of the affected muscles. Abnormal muscle ultrasound images were found in

96% of these IRU at the same location demonstrating the excellent correlation between both imaging modalities.[24] On transverse ultrasound images, affected muscle parts most frequently presented a marbled appearance created by focal or multifocal areas of increased echogenicity compared to normal hypoechoic muscle fascicules (FIGURE 11). In longitudinal scans, these alterations were seen as linear stripes of increased echogenicity. Less frequently, muscle injuries were detected as diffuse increase in echogenicity as opposed to focal lesions. Muscle ultrasonographic abnormalities can also be found in horses with normal scintigraphic images. Positive ultrasound and negative scintigraphic muscle injuries may be explained by a fibrous healing process with muscle scarring and areas of fibrotic myopathy. Ultrasound abnormalities are mainly seen within the lumbar part of the gluteus medius muscle and less frequently the latissimus dorsi muscles of racing Thoroughbreds.

Finally, ultrasound can also be used to assess the muscle level of activity through the evaluation of its cross sectional area. Recently, Stubbs et al. (2010, 2011) have studied the multifidus muscle, which plays a major role in axial stabilization and proprioception. These authors have shown that pathological changes of the spine are associated with measurable left/right asymmetry in the multifidus at or close to the level of injury. They have also observed that regular dynamic voluntary axial mobilization over a 3-month period induced hypertrophy of the multifidus muscles and increased symmetry between the left and right muscle cross sectional areas.

Conclusions

Radiography, ultrasound and scintigraphy represent complementary imaging modalities for investigating back disorders and associated axial pain in horses. With this approach the differential diagnosis of traumatic, degenerative and stress back lesions, such as kissing spines, osteoarthrosis of SIVA, spondylosis as well as soft tissue injuries can be made. Objective data are obtained allowing a better prognosis and new therapeutic approaches for equine back lesions. Finally, ultrasound has recently found some therapeutic application through the development of ultrasound guided injections and the evaluation of the effects of physiotherapy on back muscles.

Acknowledgments

The authors thank the Conseil Régional de Basse-Normandie and the European Parliament (European Regional Development Funds—FEDER) for their financial support, the Hippolia Fundation for its technical assistance and the referring veterinarians providing the cases.

References

1.   Audigié F, Didierlaurent D, Carnicer D, Denoix J-M. Examen radiographique du dos chez le cheval. *Pratique Vétérinaire Equine*. 2008;**40**:55-61.

2.   Denoix J-M. Diagnosis of the cause of back pain in horses. *Proceedings of the Conference on Equine Sports, Medicine and Science*. Córdoba. 1998. 97.

3.   Denoix J-M. Lesions of the vertebral column in poor performance horses. *Proceedings of the World Equine Veterinary Association Symposium*. 1999. 99-107.

4.   Berner D, Winter K, Brehm W, Gerlach K. Influence of head and neck position on radiographic measurement of intervertebral distances between thoracic dorsal spinous processes in clinically sound horses. *Equine Vet J*. 2012;**44**:21-26.

5.   Butler JA, Colles CM, Dyson SJ, Kold SE, Poulos PW. The spine. *Clinical Radiology of the Horse*. 3rd ed. Oxford, UK: Wiley-Blackwell; 2008;505-572.

6.   Denoix J-M. Ligament injuries of the axial skeleton in the horse: supraspinal and sacroiliac desmopathies. *Proceedings of the First Dubai International Equine Symposium*. 1996. 273-286.

7.   Denoix J-M. Ultrasonographic evaluation of back lesions. *Vet Clin North Am Equine Pract*. 1999;**15**:131-159.

8.   Fuglbjerg V, Nielsen J, Thomsen PD, Berg LC. Accuracy of ultrasound guided injections of thoracolumbar articular process joints in horses: A cadaveric study. *Equine Vet J*. 2010;**42**:18-22.

9.   Henson FM, Lamas L, Knezevic S, Jeffcott LB. Ultrasonographic evaluation of the supraspinous ligament in a series of ridden and unridden horses and horses with unrelated back pathology. *BMC Vet Res*. 2007;**3**:3.

10. Jeffcott L. Conditions causing thoracolumbar pain and dysfunction in horses. *Proceedings of the annual convention of the American Association of Equine Practitioners (USA)*, 1985;285-296.

11. Jeffcott L. Disorders of the thoracolumbar spine of the horse—A survey of 443 cases. *Equine Vet J*. 1980;**12**:197-210.

12. Denoix J-M, Dyson S. Thoracolumbar spine. In: Ross, M, Dyson, S (eds.): *Diagnosis and management of lameness in the horse*. 2nd ed. St. Louis, MO: Elsevier-Saunders Company; 2011;592-605.

13. Erichsen C, Eksell P, Holm KR, Lord P, Johnston C. Relationship between scintigraphic and radiographic evaluations of spinous processes in the thoracolumbar spine in riding horses without clinical signs of back problems. *Equine Vet J*. 2004;**36**:458-465.

14. Haussler KK, Stover S, Willits N. Pathologic changes in the lumbosacral vertebrae and pelvis in Thoroughbred racehorses. *Am J Vet Res*. 1999;**60**:143-153.

15. Zimmerman M, Dyson S, Murray R. Comparison of radiographic and scintigraphic findings of the spinous processes in the equine thoracolumbar region. *Vet Radiol Ultrasound*. 2011;**52**:661-671.

16. Zimmerman M, Dyson S, Murray R. Close, impinging and overriding spinous processes in the thoracolumbar spine: the relationship between radiological and scintigraphic findings and clinical signs. *Equine Vet J*. 2012;**44**:178-184.

17. Piat P, Blond L, Spriet M, Galuppo L, Laverty S. Fractures of the withers in horses. *Equine Vet Educ*. 2012;**24**:582-588.

18. Denoix J-M. Radiographic evaluation of the articular process joints in the thoracolumbar spine of the horse. *37th British Equine Veterinary Association Congress*. Birmingham, England, 1998.

19. Girodroux M, Dyson S, Murray R. Osteoarthritis of the thoracolumbar synovial intervertebral articulations: clinical and radiographic features in 77 horses with poor performance and back pain. *Equine Vet J*. 2009;**41**:130-138.

20. Gillen A, Dyson S, Murray R. Nuclear scintigraphic assessment of the thoracolumbar synovial intervertebral articulations. *Equine Vet J*. 2009;**41**:534-540.

21. Denoix J-M. Thoracolumbar malformations or injuries and neurological manifestations. *Equine Vet Educ*. 2005;**17**:191-194.

22. Denoix J-M. Discovertebral pathology in horses. *Equine Vet Educ*. 2007;**19**:72-73.

23. Meehan L, Dyson S, Murray R. Radiographic and scintigraphic evaluation of spondylosis in the equine thoracolumbar spine: a retrospective study. *Equine Vet J*. 2009;**41**:800-807.

24. Audigié F, Didierlaurent D, Jacquet S, Coudry V, Denoix J-M. Comparison between scintigraphic and ultrasonographic assessment of muscle injuries in sport and race horses. *Vet Radiol Ultrasound*. 2009 Jan-Feb;**50**:112.

25. Davenport-Goodall CL, Ross MW. Scintigraphic abnormalities of the pelvic region in horses examined because of lameness or poor performance: 128 cases (1993-2000). *J Am Vet Med Assoc*. 2004;**224**:88-95.

4 FROM QUANTITATIVE TO NANO-COMPUTED TOMOGRAPHY: RESEARCH AND CLINICAL APPLICATIONS

Sandra Martig

University of Melbourne, Victoria, Australia & Centre for Animal Referral and Emergency, Collingwood, Victoria, Australia

The Origin of Quantitative Computed Tomography

Quantitative computed tomography (QCT), sometimes also called osteoabsorptiometry, is almost as old as clinical computed tomography (CT). The technique was developed to assess bone mineral density in people to determine their risk of suffering an osteoporotic fracture. This article explains the principles of QCT, touches on its development beyond clinical scanners, and outlines some of the many applications. Adams' review article about QCT and osteoporosis in humans provides a great summary source of information and is recommended to the interested reader.[1]

A standard clinical scanner is used for QCT, and a phantom is scanned together with the patient. The phantom contains a hydroxyapatite equivalent of two or more known concentrations. Dedicated software converts the Hounsfield Units to the known hydroxyapatite concentrations of the phantom and calculates a conversion curve for the patient data. Central QCT refers to bone mineral density measurements of vertebral bodies, usually L1 to L3. Bone mineral density is measured in a standardised region of interest that only includes cancellous bone.[1] Peripheral QCT (pQCT) refers to assessment of a few centimetres of bone of either radius or tibia. Here total and trabecular bone mineral density measurements are often complemented by geometrical measurements including but not limited to cross-sectional area and periosteal and endosteal circumferences.[1] Radiation doses to the patient are higher with central than with peripheral QCT. Several reasons account for the currently low clinical use of QCT in human medicine: the preference to use clinical scanners for clinical purposes rather than osteoporosis screening, the high radiation doses associated with the (central) scans and the lack of mobility of the scanners. Dual energy x-ray absorptiometry (DEXA) was developed to alleviate these problems and is now predominantly used for osteoporosis screening and staging.[2] The World Health Organisation currently defines osteoporosis based on DEXA scores, which explains the widespread use of the technique.

There are, however, major differences between DEXA and QCT. Like radiography, DEXA is influenced by superimposition of structures and assesses an area of bone mineral density that includes both the cortical and trabecular bone. The cross-sectional nature of QCT allows evaluation of cortical and trabecular bone density separately. Furthermore, QCT provides information about the bone's architecture that is not available through DEXA. Cortical and trabecular architecture contribute to bone strength and fracture resistance relatively independently of bone mineral density.[3-5] Therefore research interest in cross-sectional imaging of bone persists. Dedicated pQCT and high resolution pQCT (HR-pQCT) units have been developed to circumvent the limited access to clinical scanners, reduce radiation dose to the patient and increase image resolution. These units have a small gantry that is designed to accommodate a human distal limb only and have lower maximum kilovoltage output than clinical scanners. Radiation dose to the patient is lower with pQCT and HR-pQCT machines than with peripheral scans acquired on a clinical machine.

The Race to the Highest Spatial Resolution

The main factor that determines the nomenclature from QCT all the way to nano-CT is spatial image resolution. However, not all manufacturers provide information on the modulation transfer function (MTF) to describe the spatial resolution of their system. Often the in-plane voxel size is the only information provided. Voxel size is always smaller than spatial resolution. Voxel size for pQCT using a clinical CT or a dedicated pQCT scanner is between 0.2 and 0.8 mm (i.e. 200 to 800 µm) while it is around 0.08 mm (i.e. 80 µm) using a HR-pQCT scanner (FIGURE 1). Micro-CT refers to voxel sizes between 0.001 and 0.1 mm (i.e. 1 µm to 100 µm) and nano-CT to voxel sizes in the range of nanometres (less than 0.001 mm). Voxel size should be no bigger than half the size of the structure of interest. Human trabecular bone thickness is around 0.1 to 0.2 mm (i.e. 100 to 200 µm).

The size of the specimen that can be imaged and the available field of view decrease with increasing spatial resolution. Peripheral QCT and HR-pQCT units are designed for a human distal limb and accommodate similarly sized specimens although some creativity may be required to ensure stable positioning of the specimen in the gantry. Micro-CT units can be divided into *in vivo* and *ex vivo* units. The *in/ex vivo* categorization refers to rodents, mostly mice or

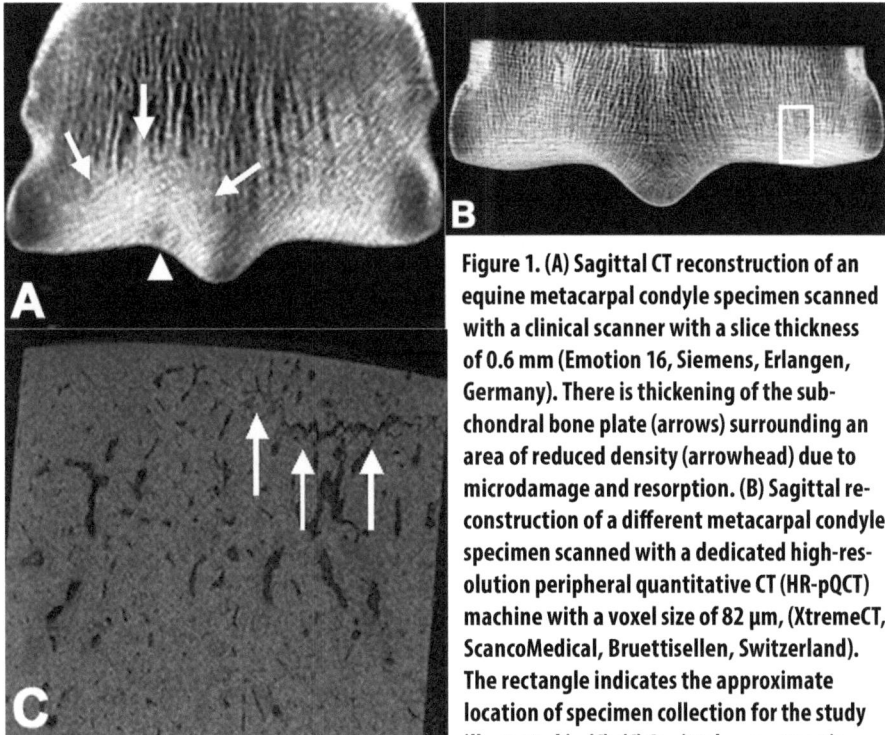

Figure 1. (A) Sagittal CT reconstruction of an equine metacarpal condyle specimen scanned with a clinical scanner with a slice thickness of 0.6 mm (Emotion 16, Siemens, Erlangen, Germany). There is thickening of the subchondral bone plate (arrows) surrounding an area of reduced density (arrowhead) due to microdamage and resorption. **(B)** Sagittal reconstruction of a different metacarpal condyle specimen scanned with a dedicated high-resolution peripheral quantitative CT (HR-pQCT) machine with a voxel size of 82 µm, (XtremeCT, ScancoMedical, Bruettisellen, Switzerland). The rectangle indicates the approximate location of specimen collection for the study illustrated in (C). **(C)** Sagittal reconstruction of a specimen sampled from a different horse at the location indicated in (B) and scanned with an *ex vivo* micro-CT machine with a nominal voxel size of 4.8 µm (Skyscan 1172, Bruker-microCT N.V., Kontich, Belgium). Microscopically small cracks (microcracks) are located parallel to the articular surface (arrows). Images (A) and (B) courtesy of Chris Whitton, Equine Centre, University of Melbourne, Australia.

rats. *In vivo* units usually provide lower spatial resolution than *ex vivo* units but are able to image larger specimens. Most units provide a range of voxel sizes to choose from. The field of view decreases with decreasing voxel size. A nano-CT scanner that resolves structures as small as osteocyte lacunae may only have a field of view of 2x2 mm. As with clinical CT scanners, image quality decreases if the object is not entirely included in the scan field of view. Therefore, only minute specimens can be imaged with a nano-CT unit.

Scanners and Image Processing

Many micro-CT machines at the higher end of resolution are *ex vivo* scanners. Their x-ray tube and detector are stationary with a horizontal beam while the specimen holder turns around its own axis (FIGURE 2). *In vivo* micro-CT machines cater to the examination of anaesthetised mice and rats. These machines provide a cradle for the rodents and have a rotating x-ray tube/detector unit similar to clinical scanners. They are often equipped with animal monitoring systems and possibly a heater, although the heat produced at the anode also contributes to warming the imaging chamber to above room temperature.

Radiation dose increases by a factor of four with increasing resolution. This may be an issue for live rodents in longitudinal studies because of the risk of radiation injuries and for dead specimens intended to undergo subsequent mechanical testing because radiation exposure may alter mechanical properties. The machines themselves are fully lead shielded (resulting in about 250 kg of weight) to eliminate radiation exposure to the operator. Micro-CT scanners can therefore be installed in any room in which the floor is designed to support the high load over a small surface area (FIGURE 2).

Micro-CT units use a 'conventional' x-ray tube with an unconventionally small focal spot of 2-5 µm in diameter (micro focus). Some nano-CT units still operate with a conventional x-ray tube while others use synchrotron light, which provides a monochromatic x-ray beam.

The small focal spot reduces penumbral blurring and enables optimal use of geometric magnification, i.e. the object is placed as close to the x-ray tube as possible while still entirely within the cone of the x-ray beam. Consequently the specimen-detector distance increases resulting in a magnified projection of the specimen.

Most micro-CT scanners work with a cone-beam (as opposed to a fan-beam) and use a charge-coupled device (CCD) as x-ray detector. Scan settings, e.g. object-detector distance, exposure parameters and beam filtering at the tube, are determined for each experiment by scanning a representative specimen with a variety of different settings and then using the best setting for all specimens of the experiment. Scan time is a function of specimen size and density and varies widely from several minutes to many hours per specimen. Phantoms are treated like an additional experimental specimen instead of being scanned together with each specimen.

Raw-data often consist of tiff images (the radiographic projections), which are reconstructed into cross-sectional images using filtered back projection. Additional post-processing filters are routinely applied during the back projection to correct for defective detector pixels and artefacts such as beam hardening artefacts and ring artefacts. As for the scan settings, these post-processing steps are optimised subjectively through trial and error based on an example specimen and should remain unchanged throughout the experiment. The filtered back projection is usually performed with proprietary software, often on the acquisition console but some manufacturers provide reconstruction software that can be installed on remote computers.

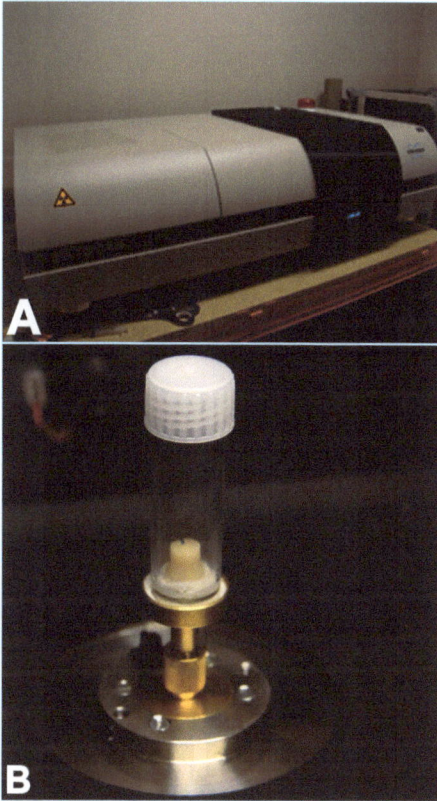

Figure 2. (A) Example of an ex-vivo tabletop micro-CT unit, Skyscan 1172 (Bruker-microCT N.V., Kontich, Belgium). The machine is fully lead shielded and radiation outside the machine is at background level at all times. (B) Bone specimen in a serum tube mounted on the specimen holder of (A). The specimen holder is a piece of precision engineering that turns around its axis with minimal wobble. The bone specimen is 7 mm long and has a diameter of 6.5 mm. A drop of saline was added to the tube to prevent drying of the bone during the scan. The condensation in the tube is due to the heat from the anode that is partially transferred to the specimen chamber. Images courtesy of Chris Whitton, Equine Centre, University of Melbourne, Australia.

The reconstructed cross-sectional images often require segmentation into two phases—for bone, these are mineralised tissue and marrow space—before the final analyses are performed. Bone analyses routinely include bone mineral density and a variety of morphometric parameters including but not limited to cortical thickness and area, the percentage of trabecular bone in the area of investigation, and trabecular number, thickness and spacing. Before the invention of micro-CT these measurements have been performed on histological sections of the area of interest, a process called histomorphometry. Bone histomorphometry is a strictly two-dimensional process where measurements and counts are acquired on a defined cross-section. The 2D values are then extrapolated into the third dimension using mathematical formulae. Micro-CT not only enables direct measurement of these indices in the three dimensional space but is also non-destructive. Experimental animals can be examined more than once during a study and *ex vivo* specimens can be used for further investigations such as mechanical testing to compare morphometric parameters with bone strength.

Computing power quickly becomes a limiting factor. For example a scan of a 5 mm long bone cylinder with a diameter of 7 mm scanned with a 4.8 µm in-plane voxel size results in approximately 1200 slices corresponding to 2 GB of

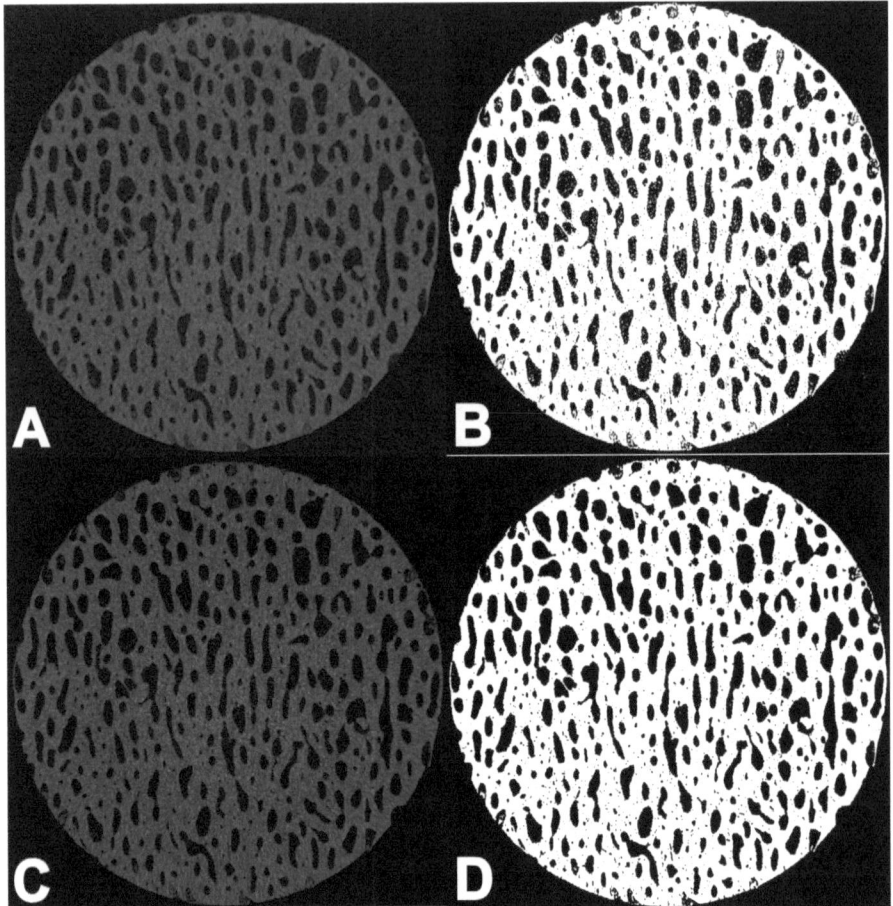

Figure 3. Examples of the influence of image processing on micro-CT images. (A) Raw cross-sectional image reconstructed from the initial radiographic projection using filters to reduce beam hardening and ring artefacts. Image noise is visible in the marrow spaces as high-density pixels and in the mineralised bone as low-density pixels. (B) Binary segmentation of the image in (A) was required for further analyses for example to determine the amount of mineralised bone (bone volume fraction) or trabecular thickness. White pixels in the marrow spaces will be counted as mineralised bone and black pixels in the mineralised bone as non-mineralised bone. (C) Same image as in (A) after smoothing and manual adjustment of contrast to reduce the visible noise in the marrow spaces. (D) The segmented binary image resulting from (C). Bone volume fraction determined from (D) will be lower than if determined from (B).

raw data for a single specimen, excluding the cross-sectional reconstructions and any further processed images.

Many manufacturers use proprietary image descriptions and software leading to incompatibility between systems similar to the situation in clinical radiology before the invention of the DICOM standard. Many researchers use open source software for image analysis not only for financial reasons but also to write their own codes for the analyses as custom software may not perform the desired analyses and the manufacturers of custom software do not always disclose their codes (FIGURE 3).

Applications: From Material Science to Double Contrast Studies of Lung Tumours in Mice

Describing non-medical micro-CT applications in detail is beyond the scope of this overview. I briefly mention some examples of micro-CT use that appear less abstract than material and soil science, two areas that commonly use micro-CT, before elaborating more on medical and veterinary applications. Micro-CT analysis of fossil teeth helped in the description of a new species of great ape (a possible human predecessor).[6] The authors suggest that the ape fed on a fibre rich diet based on the micro-CT appearance of the enamel-dentin junction, which helped them differentiate the new species from others. Micro-CT is also used in the development of new drugs. Pore size in matrix-type drug delivery systems is related to drug release rate. Different manufacturing processes result in different pore sizes and distribution. Micro-CT is an excellent tool for non-destructively assessing pore size and distribution.[7] Admittedly, this sounds much like material science, and I will move closer to the medical field.

Biomedical Engineering

Micro-CT is a useful complimentary method to histology and mechanical testing to assess osteointegration of a variety of materials ranging from metallic implants with new surface coatings over bioscaffolds to bone grafts.[8-10] Another, somewhat more abstract but growing area is computer modelling of various biological processes. The high-resolution anatomical data generated by micro-CT allows development of more refined finite element models. Such models are valuable to explore the (expected) strength of a structure and how the structure may respond to different environments. Both clinical and micro-CT scanners have been used to provide input into finite element models of equine gait.[11,12] It is impossible to measure joint surface pressure and bone strain *in vivo* without altering joint and bones and therefore the stresses they experience. Finite element models enable calculation of the forces that act on the joint surface and within the bones. Such models could, for example, be used to provide guidance for optimizing training regimes once the biological response of the bone to these stresses can be incorporated.

In addition to the anatomical information, finite element models also require input on the material properties, for example stiffness, of the structure under investigation. The non-destructive nature of micro-CT enables subsequent mechanical testing of the same specimen to determine its mechanical properties. For example, stiffness of the periodontal ligament of equine teeth is a required input variable for finite element analysis of the effect of mastication on teeth.[13,14] Finite element modelling then enables the investigation of different patterns of mastication, the effect of different feed types on mastication and the resulting forces on the teeth and their effect on dental health.

Basic and Clinical Research in Human Disease

Osteoporosis is one of the biggest areas of basic bone research. Researchers investigate the molecular steps of and factors involved in bone resorption and production in order to find new drug targets for the treatment or prevention of osteoporosis. The effect of knockout genes, ovariectomy (allegedly mimicking menopause) or antiresorptive drug candidates were historically assessed through bone histomorphometry after sacrifice of the experimental animals. Micro-CT enables longitudinal studies where mice are imaged *in vivo* to assess bone mineral density and trabecular architecture. Even if the classic study design remains unchanged, micro-CT analysis of the bones *ex vivo* provides a more accurate assessment of the three dimensional structure than the two dimensional histomorphometry.

Micro-CT has also found its way into clinical research. The technique is used to assess human bone biopsies either alone or in conjunction with other methods. For example, Huang and co-workers examined biopsies to assess the osteointegration of bone grafts that were implanted into sinuses of people who required a maxillary dental implant but had not enough bone available to anchor the implant.[15]

Soft Tissue Micro-CT

Like clinical CT, micro-CT often relies on contrast medium injection for soft tissue imaging. Mice models of cerebro- and cardiovascular diseases require some thinking outside the box to find the ideal site of contrast medium injection. The tail vein is a standard injection site in rodents but such injections resulted in poor cardiac contrast while a bolus injection into the retrobulbar sinus provided good contrast filling of the heart.[16] Ashton and co-workers used two contrast media (gold nanoparticles and liposomal iodine) for imaging of a murine lung tumour model with a custom built dual-energy micro-CT scanner.[17] They even used respiratory gating to reduce motion artefacts. However, the authors mention that sub-voxel size motion (e.g. from cardiac motion) still affected image quality and their ability to accurately measure tumour size, which in this feasibility study was sometimes less than 1 mm in diameter.

What Is Happening in the Veterinary Field?

Restrictions in specimen size and high equipment costs have so far limited the use of micro-CT in the veterinary field. The following is a brief overview of current veterinary related literature that includes the use of QCT in some form. This overview is not intended to be complete, and some applications may have been overlooked.

Veterinary In Vivo Applications

A single case report described the use of an *in vivo* rodent micro-CT machine (MicroCAT II, Siemens) instead of a clinical CT unit to scan the head of a client owned guinea pig with exophthalmos and strabismus.[18] Images were acquired with an isotropic voxel size of 0.077 mm. A diagnosis of a periapical tooth abscess and adjacent osteomyelitis was made, and the guinea pig responded favourably to a prolonged course of antibiotics.

De Rycke and co-workers published a high resolution CT atlas of the rabbit head based on micro-CT images with an isotropic voxel size of 0.055 mm.[19] This atlas is of great value for clinicians albeit vexing as the resolution of clinical images is far from the images in the atlas.

Anaesthetised live research horses were examined on several occasions with a pQCT scanner (XCT 2000, Stratec, Pforzheim, Germany) in a longitudinal study on the effect of detraining on the bones of racehorses. Sections of the diaphysis and the distal epiphysis of a metacarpal bone were scanned and assessed for bone mineral density, bone area, cortical circumferences and their effect on bone strength immediately before and after eight months of training and after 4.5 months of detraining.[20]

The authors of a *post mortem* study on the effect of age on bones in horses mention that it may be technically possible to examine the distal phalanx of anaesthetized live horses with the HR-pQCT unit they used (XtremeCT Scanco Medical, Bruettisellen, Switzerland), enabling voxel sizes between 0.04 and 0.246 mm (FIGURE 4).[21]

In veterinary dentistry, grafts are more commonly used to fill defects after tooth extraction rather than to prepare the socket for a dental implant. Vlaminck and co-workers examined biopsies with micro-CT to assess the osteointegration of a non resorbable bone substitute after tooth extraction in ponies.[22] The core biopsies were collected with a trephine burr twelve months after tooth extraction and were assessed with micro-CT and histologically. The study continued beyond the 12 months, demonstrating the potential of micro-CT to be integrated into longitudinal *in vivo* studies.

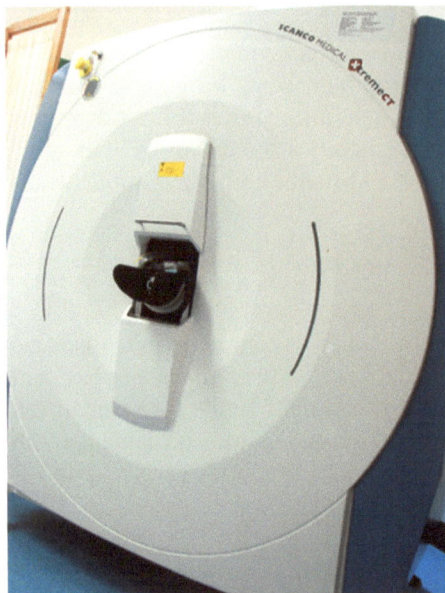

Figure 4. Example of a dedicated high-resolution peripheral quantitative CT (HR-pQCT) machine, XtremeCT (ScancoMedical, Bruettisellen, Switzerland). The plastic bag in the gantry contains a bone specimen cut from an equine metacarpal condyle. The height above ground of the gantry is designed for a person to comfortably sit in a chair and hold a hand or foot into the gantry to scan the distal aspect of the forearm or lower leg, respectively. Image courtesy of Chris Whitton, Equine Centre, University of Melbourne, Australia.

Ex Vivo Basic Bone Research

Quantitative and micro-CT have mostly been used to investigate two conditions in veterinary medicine: canine elbow dysplasia (mainly fragmented medial coronoid process) and subchondral bone injuries in the metacarpal condyles and carpal bones of racehorses. Quantitative CT evaluation of radiographically normal canine elbow joints has been described over a decade ago.[23] Computer power was a limiting factor at the time and together with limited machine and software availability may be part of the reason while it took almost ten years for quantitative CT to resurface in the literature on canine elbow dysplasia. Dickomeit and co-workers investigated the subchondral bone density of the entire articular surface of normal elbow joints and developed surface density maps as a function of age.[24] Both research groups used cadaver limbs, most likely for logistical purposes and study design (e.g. normal cartilage on visual inspection as inclusion criterion) rather than scanner limitations. Quantitative CT is possible in live dogs in a clinical setting if the elbows are scanned together with a phantom and the required software is available. Longitudinal studies and comparison of normal and abnormal elbows are required to further evaluate the usefulness of QCT for investigation of the canine elbow dysplasia complex for research, screening and clinical purposes.

Wolschrjin and Wim investigated at what age the subchondral bone of the medial coronoid process of Golden Retrievers puppies changed from a porous trabecular structure to a solid closed plate.[25] The puppies were euthanised at different ages, and specimens of the medial coronoid process were examined both with micro-CT and histology. The same group also used micro-CT in addition to necropsy as a gold standard for final diagnosis of medial coronoid disease vs. normal in another experiment.[26]

In equine research, micro-CT and p-QCT offer many possibilities to investigate normal anatomy and the subchondral bone's response to training.[27-31] An HR-pQCT unit (XtremeCT, Scanco Medical, Bassersdorf, Switzerland) was used to investigate bone remodelling and metacarpal condylar fractures in *post mortem* specimens of Thoroughbred racehorses.[32] A clinical scanner was used to perform QCT on *post mortem* specimens in a study on how exercise early in a foal's life affects bone.[33]

Different Ways of Using Contrast Media to Assess Cartilage with Micro-CT

Like clinical CT, micro-CT relies on contrast medium application for cartilage visualisation. Air adjacent to the cartilage may be sufficient as contrast medium to allow measurement of cartilage thickness. However, more sophisticated contrast procedures have been developed. Equilibrium partitioning of an ionic contrast agent with micro-CT (EPIC-micro-CT) specifically uses the negative charge of the iodine-carrying molecules in ionic contrast media to determine the proteoglycan content of cartilage.[34] The cartilage specimens are immersed in contrast medium solution for staining. The negatively charged iodine carrying molecules accumulate in areas of cartilage with low proteoglycan content because proteoglycans are also negatively charged. The correlation between the concentrations of contrast medium and proteoglycans in cartilage is linear (and inverse, i.e. the more proteoglycans, the less contrast medium). Lau and co-workers used this technique in canine medial coronoid process specimens and demonstrated statistically significant higher contrast medium uptake in the cartilage of specimens with bony fissures or fragments compared to specimens without fissures or fragments.[35]

A *post mortem* perfusion technique was used to investigate osteochondrosis in the tarsus of Standardbred foals.[36] Micronized barium sulfate was injected into the femoral artery immediately after euthanasia to fill the arterial side of circulation. Seven out of eight early osteochondrosis lesions found on histologic examination were seen on micro-CT as areas of growth cartilage without detectable arterial perfusion. Focal defects in the subchondral bone plate were also present in some of these lesions.

Summary

Quantitative CT refers to the measurement of bone mineral density by converting Hounsfield Units of bone into bone mineral density in g/cm³ based on the comparison with a phantom of known hydroxyapatite concentrations. The names of the various quantitative CT methods are derived from the voxel size they achieve: clinical and pQCT scanners have voxel sizes in the range of

0.2 to 0.8 mm, micro-CT in the range of micrometres (0.001 to 0.1 mm), and nano-CT in the range of nanometers (< 0.001 mm). Micro-CT is used by many different disciplines including, but not limited to soil science, pharmacology, biomedical engineering and basic medical research. The abilities of micro-CT are currently explored in veterinary research to elucidate the pathophysiology of canine medial coronoid disease, equine subchondral bone injuries and equine dental disease. Veterinary clinical application of micro-CT is currently limited to small pets using facilities developed for research rodents. However, the future for clinical use is exciting: with increasing availability of clinical CT scanners the potential of QCT should be explored further, pQCT scanners could be used for larger animals *in vivo* and micro-CT has great potential to complement traditional histology in the analysis of bone biopsies.

References

1.   Adams JE. Quantitative computed tomography. *Eur J Radiol.* 2009;**71**: 415-424.

2.   Kanis JA, Delmas P, Burckhardt P, Cooper C, Torgerson D. Guidelines for diagnosis and management of osteoporosis. *Osteoporosis Int.* 1997;7:390-406.

3.   Goldstein SA. The mechanical properties of trabecular bone: dependence on anatomic location and function. *J Biomech.* 1987;**20**:1055-1061.

4.   Rho JY, Kuhn-Spearing L, Zioupos P. Mechanical properties and the hierarchical structure of bone. *Med Eng & Phys.* 1998;**20**:92-102.

5.   Martin RB, Burr DB, Sharkey NA. Mechanical Properties of Bone. *Skeletal Tissue Mechanics.* New York: Springer, 2010.

6.   Suwa G, Kono RT, Katoh S, Asfaw B, Beyene Y. A new species of great ape from the late Miocene epoch in Ethiopia. *Nature.* 2007;**448**:921-924.

7.   Wang Y, Wertheim DF, Jones AS, Chang H-I, Coombes AGA. Micro-CT Analysis of Matrix-Type Drug Delivery Devices and Correlation With Protein Release Behaviour. *J Pharm Sci.* 2010;**99**:2854-2862.

8.   Fang L, Ding X, Wang H-m, Zhu X-H. Chronological changes in the microstructure of bone during peri-implant healing: a microcomputed tomographic evaluation. *Brit J Oral Max Surg.* 2014;**52**:816-821.

9.   Hong J-Y, Kang S-W, Kim J-W, Suh S-W, Ko Y-J, Park J-H. Optimal condition of heparin-conjugated fibrin with bone morphogenetic protein-2 for spinal fusion in a rabbit model. *Cytotherapy.* 2014;**16**:1441-1448.

10. Toda M, Ohno J, Shinozaki Y, Ozaki M, Fukushima T. Osteogenic potential for replacing cells in rat cranial defects implanted with a DNA/protamine complex paste. *Bone.* 2014;**67**:237-245.

11. O'Hare LMS, Cox PG, Jeffery N, Singer ER. Finite element analysis of stress in the equine proximal phalanx. *Equine Vet J*. 2013;**45**:273-277.

12. Harrison SM, Whitton RC, Kawcak CE, Stover SM, Pandy MG. Evaluation of a subject-specific finite-element model of the equine metacarpophalangeal joint under physiological load. *J Biomech*. 2013.

13. Lupke M, Gardemin M, Kopke S, Seifert H, Staszyk C. Finite element analysis of the equine periodontal ligament under masticatory loading. *Wien Tierarz Monats*. 2010;**97**:101-106.

14. Schrock P, Luepke M, Seifert H, Borchers L, Staszyk C. Finite element analysis of equine incisor teeth. Part 1: Determination of the material parameters of the periodontal ligament. *Vet J*. 2013;**198**:583-589.

15. Huang H-L, Chen MYC, Hsu J-T, Li Y-F, Chang C-H, Chen K-T. Three-dimensional bone structure and bone mineral density evaluations of autogenous bone graft after sinus augmentation: a microcomputed tomography analysis. *Clin Oral Implan Res*. 2012;**23**:1098-1103.

16. Socher M, Kuntz J, Sawall S, Bartling S, Kachelriess M. The retrobulbar sinus is superior to the lateral tail vein for the injection of contrast media in small animal cardiac imaging. *Lab Anim*. 2014;**48**:105-113.

17. Ashton JR, Clark DP, Moding EJ, Ghaghada K, Kirsch DG, West JL, et al. Dual-Energy Micro-CT Functional Imaging of Primary Lung Cancer in Mice Using Gold and Iodine Nanoparticle Contrast Agents: A Validation Study. *Plos One*. 2014;**9**:e88129.

18. Souza MJ, Greenacre CB, Avenell JS, Wall JS, Daniel GB. Diagnosing a Tooth Root Abscess in a Guinea Pig (Cavia porcellus) Using Micro Computed Tomography Imaging. *J Exot Pet Med*. 2006;**15**:274-277.

19. De Rycke LM, Boone MN, Van Caelenberg AI, Dierick M, Van Hoorebeke L, van Bree H, et al. Micro-computed tomography of the head and dentition in cadavers of clinically normal rabbits. *Am J Vet Res*. 2012;**73**:227-232.

20. Firth EC, Rogers CW, Van Weeren PR, Barneveld A, Kawcak CE, McIlwraith CW, et al. Changes in diaphyseal and epiphyseal bone parameters in thoroughbred horses after withdrawal from training. *J Musculoskelet Neuronal Interact*. 2007;7:74-76.

21. Fuerst A, Meier D, Michel S, Schmidlin A, Held L, Laib A. Effect of age on bone mineral density and micro architecture in the radius and tibia of horses: An Xtreme computed tomographic study. *BMC Vet Res*. 2008;**4**:3.

22. Vlaminck L, Cnudde V, Pieters K, Van Den Broeck W, Steenhaut M, Jacobs P, et al. Histologic and micro-computed tomographic evelution of the osseointegration of a nonresorbable bone substitue in alveoli of ponies after tooth extraction. *Am J Vet Res*. 2008;**69**:604-610.

23. Samii VF, Les CM, Schulz KS, Keyak JH, Stover SM. Computed tomographic osteoabsorptiometry of the elbow joint in clinically normal dogs. *Am J Vet Res*. 2002;**63**:1159-1166.

24. Dickomeit MJ, Boettcher P, Hecht S, Liebich H-G, Maierl J. Topographic and age-dependent distribution of subchondral bone density in the elbow joints of clinically normal dogs. *Am J Vet Res*. 2011;**72**:491-499.

25. Wolschrijn CF, Weijs WA. Development of the subchondral bone layer of the medial coronoid process of the canine ulna. *Anat Rec Part A*. 2005;**284A**:439-445.

26. Lau SF, Wolschrijn CF, Hazewinkel HAW, Siebelt M, Voorhout G. The early development of medial coronoid disease in growing Labrador retrievers: Radiographic, computed tomographic, necropsy and micro-computed tomographic findings. *Vet J*. 2013;**197**:724-730.

27. Rubio-Martinez LM, Cruz AM, Gordon K, Hurtig MB. Structural characterization of subchondral bone in the distal aspect of third metacarpal bones from Thoroughbred racehorses via micro-computed tomography. *Am J Vet Res*. 2008;**69**:1413-1422.

28. Leahy PD, Smith BS, Easton KL, Kawcak CE, Eickhoff JC, Shetye SS, et al. Correlation of mechanical properties within the equine third metacarpal with trabecular bending and multi-density micro-computed tomography data. *Bone*. 2010;**46**:1108-1113.

29. Firth EC, Rogers CW, Doube M, Jopson NB. Musculoskeletal responses of 2-year-old Thoroughbred horses to early training. 6. Bone parameters in the third metacarpal and third metatarsal bones. *N Z Vet J*. 2005;**53**:101-112.

30. Firth EC, Rogers CW. Musculoskeletal responses of 2-year-old Thoroughbred horses to early training. 7. Bone and articular cartilage response in the carpus. *N Z Vet J*. 2005;**53**:113-122.

31. Brama PAJ, Firth EC, van Weeren PR, Tuukkanen J, Holopainen J, Helminen HJ, et al. Influence of intensity and changes of physical activity on bone mineral density of immature equine subchondral bone. *Equine Vet J*. 2009;**41**:564-571.

32. Whitton RC, Trope GD, Ghasem-Zadeh A, Anderson GA, Parkin TDH, Mackie EJ, et al. Third metacarpal condylar fatigue fractures in equine athletes occur within previously modelled subchondral bone. *Bone*. 2010;**47**:826-831.

33. Kawcak CE, McIlwraith CW, Firth EC. Effects of early exercise on metacarpophalangeal joints in horses. *Am J Vet Res*. 2010;**71**:405-411.

34. Palmer AW, Guldberg RE, Levenston ME. Analysis of cartilage matrix fixed charge density and three-dimensional morphology via contrast-enhanced microcomputed tomography. *P Natl Acad Sci USA*. 2006;**103**:19255-19260.

35. Lau SF, Wolschrijn CF, Siebelt M, Vernooij JCM, Voorhout G, Hazewinkel HAW. Assessment of articular cartilage and subchondral bone using EPIC-microCT in Labrador retrievers with incipient medial coronoid disease. *Vet J.* 2013;**198**:116-121.

36. Olstad K, Cnudde V, Masschaele B, Thomassen R, Dolvik NI. Micro-computed tomography of early lesions of osteochondrosis in the tarsus of foals. *Bone.* 2008;**43**:574-583.

5 LOW-FIELD MAGNETIC RESONANCE IMAGING OF THE CANINE STIFLE JOINT

Martin Konar

MR Support Service, Marina di Massa, Italy

Abbreviations

LF MRI low-field magnetic resonance imaging (0.19-0.50 T)
HF MRI high-field magnetic resonance imaging
SNR   signal-to-noise ratio
STIR   short tau inversion recovery
IPR   in-plane resolution
FSE   fast spin echo
PD   proton density weighted
GE   gradient echo
SPGR   spoiled gradient recalled acquisition in steady state
MRA   magnetic resonance arthrography
BELL   bone marrow (o)edema like lesion
FNA   fine needle aspiration
SE   spin echo

Is Low-field Magnetic Resonance Imaging Not Keeping Its Promises for Imaging the Canine Stifle?

Sixteen years have passed since Baird et al. published two papers on the clinical application of low-field magnetic resonance imaging (LF MRI) of the canine stifle joint.[1,2] Despite all initial enthusiasm, the modality has not yet reached general acceptance for this indication.

In particular, the accuracy of the modality for evaluation of the canine menisci is discussed controversially,[3-7] with disappointing results in larger studies.[3,7] So, is LF MRI generally not capable for thorough evaluation of canine stifle joints? The author believes otherwise.

First, it is important to be aware that all published values for diagnostic accuracy are only valid for the diagnostic system used for the specific study, consisting of MRI hardware, software (protocols) and reader. They are not representative of LF MRI in general. Second, good image quality is essential for good results, and it does not come for free with the scanner. Protocol optimization requires a lot of intense work and has to be refined with every software or hardware update. Study results from images acquired with an old LF MRI system and possibly suboptimal protocols cannot be considered as "generally valid".

Third, experience is necessary. The stifle joint is complicated and includes many small structures that are visible with MRI but are only incompletely described in standard anatomy books. It takes time to learn the normal imaging anatomy.

Finally, patient size matters in LF MRI. Larger dogs, generally those weighing more than ~15 kg, typically have joint diameters that produce images of sufficient quality allowing evaluation of all relevant structures. In dogs between 10 and 15 kg, the results will heavily depend on the hardware (field strength, gradients and coil design and size). With cats and smaller dogs, cartilage will not be visible and menisci and ligaments will only rarely be able to be evaluated.

This paper, while far from covering every aspect of stifle joint MRI, intends to show what can be achieved with current LF MRI scanners.

Protocols

Image quality is essential for being able to reliably evaluate MRI studies. Tissue contrast and resolution are the main contributors to high quality images.[8] Contrast is generally considered to be good in LF MRI. The maximal achievable resolution is a direct consequence of the signal to noise ratio (SNR), which is lower in LF compared to high-field (HF) systems.

Protocols for imaging the canine stifle joint with a LF MRI system have to be designed so as to get the maximum possible resolution out of the system. This means the limits of SNR and gradient load have to be reached. If this is done, high quality images of the canine stifle joint can be achieved with a field strength as low as 0.2 T. Unfortunately, sequence parameters have to be adapted to the particular MRI unit in use, so detailed parameters can only be given as an example for one of the smaller scanners (TABLE 1).

Sequence	Plane	Repetition Time (ms)	Echo Time/ Inversion Time (ms)	Flip Angle	Field of View fe×pe†	Matrix fe×pe†	IPR‡ (mm²)	Slice thickness/ Separation (mm)	# of slices	Time (mm:ss)
GE STIR	dor	1680	25/75	90°	190×160	192×168	0.94	3/0.3	17	4:47
GE T2*	sag/dor	1395	28	65°	160×130	256×156	0.52	2.5/0.5	24	7:20
3D T1	sag	38	16	65°	180×150	192×160	0.88	1.1/0	52	6:26
TSE T2	tra	3180	100	90°	160×160	192×192	0.69	4.5/0.5	19	6:05
Total Scan time										31:57

Table 1. Example of Optimized Stifle Joint Protocol, Coil 4, VetMR, 0.19 T, Esaote, Genova, Italy

† frequency encoding × phase encoding
‡ In-plane resolution

A fat suppressing sequence has to be part of each musculoskeletal MRI exam. In LF MRI, this will usually be a short tau inversion recovery (STIR). It provides reliable fat suppression and is highly sensitive for detection of fluid but has inherently low SNR. With smaller coils, it can still be performed with 1 mm isotropic in-plane resolution (IPR) and 3 mm slice thickness, with bigger coils going up to 4 mm slice thickness. Sequence time will be between 5 and 7 minutes. It should be performed in dorsal (preferred by the author) or sagittal plane; both planes together in one exam are usually not necessary. The sequence allows for a good evaluation of muscles, bone marrow and joint fluid and will give a quick overview on the pathologic conditions of the joint. Due to its low resolution, it is of only limited use for the evaluation of ligaments and menisci.

For evaluation of menisci and ligaments, a very high-resolution sequence with good contrast is necessary. Both proton density-w fast spin echo (FSE PD-w) and T2*-w gradient echo (GE T2*-w) sequences can achieve this. Whereas a FSE PD sequence is not available on all LF MRI scanners, a GE T2*-w sequence is a standard sequence present on every MRI machine and can provide high resolution and excellent contrast for menisci and ligaments within a reasonable scan time (e.g. IPR 0.52 mm² with 2.5 mm slice thickness in 7:20 min at 0.2 T, IPR 0.35 mm² with 2 mm slice thickness in 5:54 min at 0. 25 T). This sequence has to be performed in dorsal and sagittal imaging planes in order to identify partial volume artefacts and to detect tears that are oriented parallel to the slices in one plane.

A T1-w 3D GE spoiled gradient recalled acquisition in steady state (SPGR) is also available in all LF MRI scanners. As a 3D sequence it can be performed without interslice gap and with isotropic resolution of 0.9 mm³ or even less. Due to the high resolution, other planes can be reformatted directly out of the original sequence with only mildly decreased image quality. Unfortunately, this sequence does not provide sufficient contrast for evaluating menisci and cruciate ligaments, but it is the sequence of choice for visualizing the joint cartilage.

The last sequence of the standard protocol is a transverse FSE T2-w sequence. It allows assessment of patellar position and ligaments, and the muscles of the stifle joint region. It will not help to evaluate cruciate ligaments or menisci. It should cover the area from just proximal to the patella to the proximal aspect of the tibia. Resolution is less essential, and it can be done with up to 4.5 mm slice thickness using an IPR of about 0.7 mm².

Contrast medium should be administered intravenously only if no lesion has been detected in the standard sequences or if there is a neoplastic or unclear lesion, and the 3D GE T1-w sequence should be repeated. Other sequences or alternate planes can be performed additionally but are not considered essential.

Direct and indirect MR arthrography (MRA) have shown benefits in humans,[9-11] and direct MRA has provided additional information in the canine stifle joint.[12,13] Apart from adding the risk of an invasive procedure, in the author's experience it is difficult to achieve contrast agent distribution into the region of interest and MRA may be unnecessary when using highly optimized standard protocols.

Anatomical Structures

Ligaments

Evaluation of ligaments includes assessment of delineation, course, thickness and signal intensity (hypointense in standard sequences).

Cruciate Ligaments

Stifle joint instability due to damage of the cruciate ligaments is the most common cause of osteoarthritis in the canine stifle joint.[14-17] Contrary to humans where ligament damage is most often secondary to a stifle trauma, in dogs only the rupture of the caudal cruciate ligament typically has a traumatic genesis, whereas cranial cruciate ligament rupture more commonly occurs as the result of chronic ligament damage.[15,18-25]

Joint instability increases secondary to ligament damage, resulting in more severe osteoarthritis and synovitis that further damages the cruciate ligaments.

In order to interrupt this cycle and start with early treatment, it is important to recognize cruciate ligament ruptures in a very early state of minor partial rupture. This should be a main indication for stifle joint MRI, which of course requires thorough evaluation of "mainly intact" appearing ligaments. MRI is not required to confirm the rupture of the cranial cruciate ligament if clinical signs are unequivocal but can be useful for evaluation of secondary joint damage, such as meniscal tears or cartilage lesions.

Thin slices (maximum 3 mm) should be used for imaging of the cranial cruciate ligament. With LF MRI, 2.5 mm slice thickness can be obtained at 0.2 T; at 0.25 T and higher, 2 mm are preferred. Specially dedicated planes for evaluation of the cranial cruciate ligament have been proposed,[26] but in the author's opinion this is not absolutely necessary. Mild adaption of the angle of sagittal slices demonstrates the cranial cruciate ligament within one slice (FIGURE 1) and does not impair meniscal evaluation.[13,27] The proposed oblique dorsal plane instead makes it impossible to evaluate the menisci with the same sequence, necessitating the acquisition of an additional sequence and thus prolonging examination time.

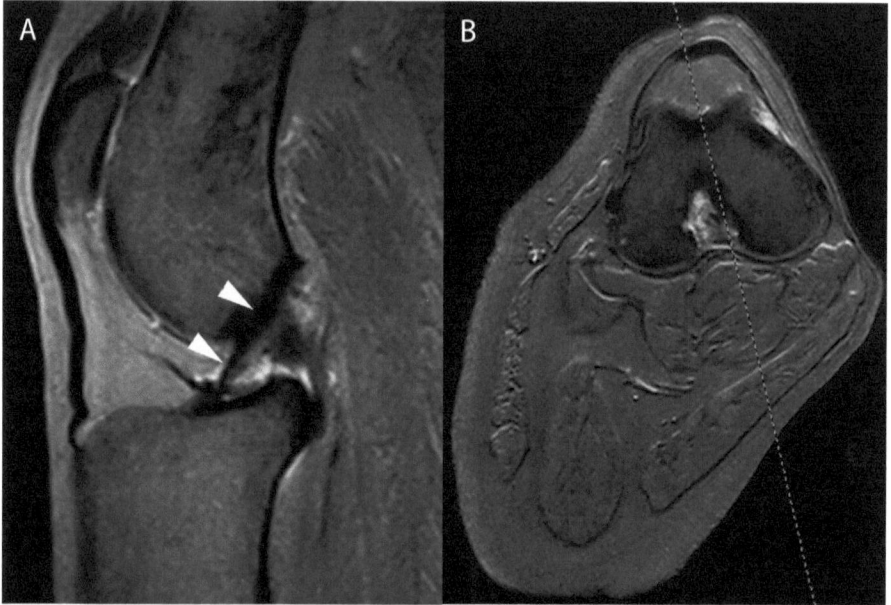

Figure 1. GE T2*-w images of the stifle of a normal 11 y F German Shepherd dog (35 kg). (A) The whole length of the cranial cruciate ligament (arrowheads) is visible in one mildly oblique sagittal slice. Cranial is to the left. (B) The exact slice orientation is shown, obliquely parallel to the axial border of the lateral femoral condyle. Lateral is to the right. (VetGrande, 0.25 T, Esaote, Genova, Italy)

In the author's experience, even with adapted slice orientation it may be difficult to evaluate a damaged cruciate ligament in a reliable way on sagittal images. Due to its torqued or even aberrant course and irregular surface and signal intensity, it may not be visible even if the main portion is still intact (Figure 3A, B). Therefore, the author prefers evaluation of both cruciate ligaments on standard dorsal plane images. Each slice will cut in a mildly oblique transverse direction through the cranial and in an oblique dorsal orientation through the caudal cruciate ligament, allowing for exact evaluation of presence, course, thickness, signal intensity and delineation of both (Figure 2). In this plane it is easily possible to follow both cruciate ligaments from their origin to their insertion. Since a standard plane is used, the menisci, the meniscofemoral ligaments and the collateral ligaments can also be evaluated concurrently. As already stated under protocols, the best combination of resolution, contrast and SNR in LF MRI is provided by the GE T2*-w or the FSE PD sequence. Normal cruciate ligaments will be easily identified in both sagittal and dorsal planes. They are sharply delineated and have expected orientation. The caudal cruciate ligament will be hypointense and mildly broader than the cranial cruciate ligament. The cranial cruciate ligament often shows mildly brighter signal intensity but maintains normal diameter and sharp delineation on each slice, in contrast to partial ruptures (Figure 2).[17,28-30]

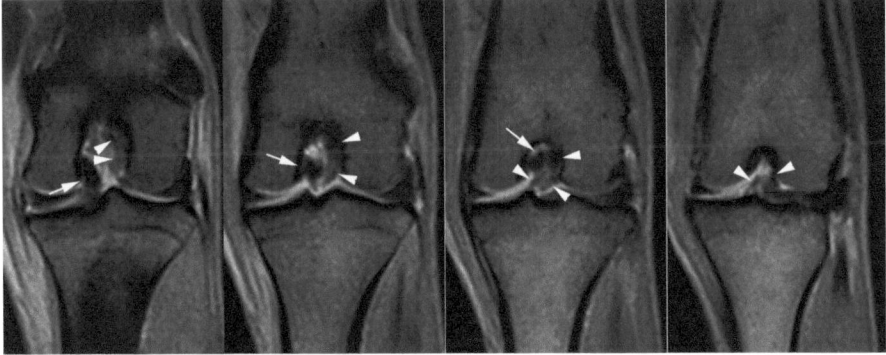

Figure 2. Consecutive dorsal GE T2*-w images of the stifle of a normal 9 y F mixed breed dog (20 kg). Images are oriented from caudal to cranial demonstrating course and delineation of normal cranial (arrowheads) and caudal (small arrows) cruciate ligaments. Note the mildly brighter signal of the cranial cruciate ligament. Lateral is to the right. (VetGrande, 0. 25 T, Esaote, Genova, Italy)

Mild partial ruptures or superficial fraying (less than ~30% of the ligament ruptured) can be difficult to identify. The signal of the ligament will be increased, often irregularly, and delineation is reduced, but the main portion of the ligament is still present and follows a normal course (Figure 3A). This is a common finding in the caudal cruciate ligament in dogs with cranial cruciate ligament ruptures.[24]

Moderate ruptures (between ~30-60% of the ligament damaged) will show significant thinning of the visible portion of the ligament. Usually on sagittal slices very little to none of the ligament is visible, whereas on dorsal images a thin portion of the ligament still follows a normal course and has only mildly changed signal (Figure 3C).

Severe partial ruptures affecting more than ~60% of the ligament can be difficult to differentiate from total ruptures. On sagittal slices the ligament usually is not visible anymore, and on dorsal slices only a few fibres will follow a normal course.

With total ruptures, the ligament will be missing in both planes (Figure 3D), but sometimes haemorrhage or fibrin can mimic a false ligament, leading to the misdiagnosis of a partial rupture. Luckily, the significantly increased signal intensity and significantly decreased delineation should still indicate at least a severe partial rupture, so proper treatment should be still be prescribed in these cases.

Secondary changes of cruciate ligament ruptures are very helpful for detecting mild partial ruptures and avulsions. Bone marrow [o]edema-like lesions (BELLs) or subchondral cysts around the origin and/or the insertion of the cranial cruciate ligament are a very common finding.[1,31,32] These should always

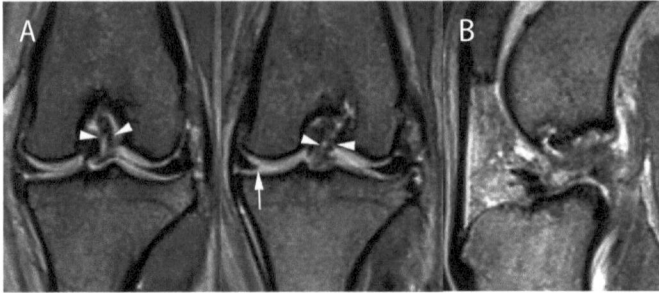

Figure 3. (A,B) GE T2*-w images of the stifle of a 2y F Broholmer dog (49 kg) with a mild partial cranial cruciate ligament tear. (A) Consecutive dorsal slices (lateral to the right) from caudal to cranial demonstrating thinning and irregular, increased signal intensity of the cranial cruciate ligament (arrowheads). (B) The sagittal slice (cranial to the left) through the expected plane of the cranial cruciate ligament does not delineate any ligament at all. Note the blunted axial tip of the medial meniscus consistent with mild axial fibrillation (A: small arrow).

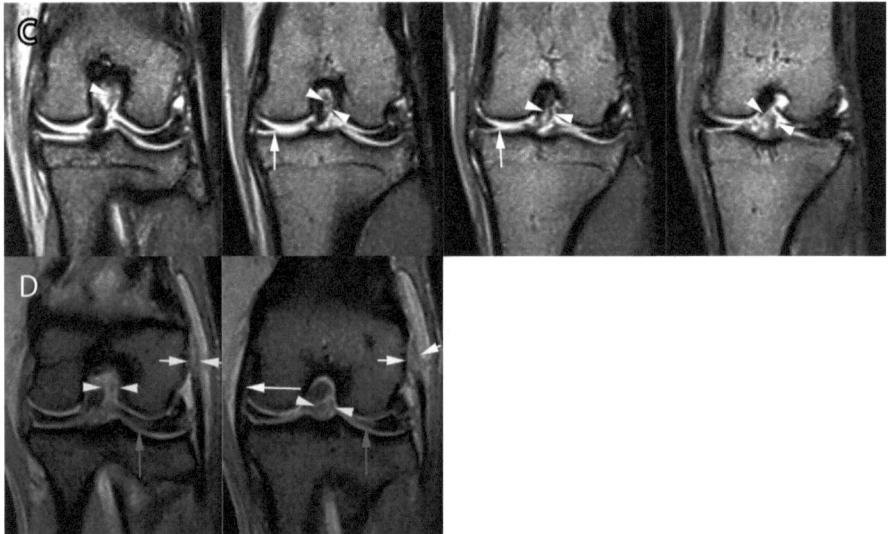

(C) GE T2*-w images of the stifle of a 2y F Rhodesian ridgeback dog (38 kg) with a moderate partial cranial cruciate ligament tear. In comparison to 3A, further thinning (to <50% of normal diameter) and increased signal of the cranial cruciate ligament (arrowheads) is present. The normal sharp axial tip of the medial meniscus is visible (arrows). (D) GE T2*-w images of the stifle of a 6 y M Flat-Coated Retriever dog (15 kg) with a complete cranial cruciate ligament tear. Dorsal consecutive slices are presented from caudal to cranial. The cranial cruciate ligament is missing (arrowheads) due to total rupture. Irregular fibres are still visible only near the insertion. Near its origin the lateral collateral ligament shows diffusely increased signal intensity (small arrows, compare with medial collateral ligament – large arrow) consistent with grade one ligament sprain. The axial parts of the body and caudal horn of the lateral meniscus show mild and diffuse hyperintense signal, typical for meniscal degeneration. (VetGrande, 0. 25 T, Esaote, Genova, Italy)

be considered as an indication for possible cruciate ligament damage ("alarm BELLs"). In cases with primary osteoarthritis, they can be the first sign of early cruciate ligament damage.

Avulsion of cruciate ligaments can be diagnosed on radiographs, and careful evaluation of bony contours will allow detection on MRI. Small fragments of bone, however, can be very easily missed since they can have the same signal intensity as ligaments or joint capsule.

If the cruciate ligaments appear intact or only mildly damaged in a joint with significant joint effusion or osteoarthritis, causes other than primary cruciate ligament disease should be considered as the reason for joint pathology.

Meniscofemoral Ligament

The meniscofemoral ligament is usually best seen on dorsal plane images, where it can be followed as an oblique hypointense structure leading from the most axial border of the caudal horn of the lateral meniscus to the axial caudal border of the medial femoral condyle. On sagittal slices it can be seen as a small round hypointense structure passing the intercondylar area caudally to the cranial cruciate ligament and proximally to the caudal cruciate ligament.

Lesions of the meniscofemoral ligament are rare. It appears that the caudal horn of the lateral meniscus ruptures rather than the ligament itself. This should mainly be considered when the meniscofemoral ligament follows a steeper course than usual.

Collateral Ligaments

Significant lesions of the collateral ligaments are rarely seen in MRI. This may be partly due to the easy clinical diagnosis of a total ligament rupture.

The ligaments can be best evaluated in the dorsal plane. Additionally, the transverse plane can help to assess ligament thickness or unclear findings in the dorsal plane. The GE T2*-w sequence or the FSE PD sequence are most useful for evaluating the collateral ligaments. The transverse FSE T2-w sequence helps in evaluating contour and thickness. The STIR sequence will only show more severe lesions but is very helpful for detection of bone marrow changes at the attachment sites.

Normal ligaments will be hypointense and sharply defined in all sequences. Ligament lesions have been graded as sprain injuries, from grade 1 (normal course, delineation and thickness; mildly increased signal intensity and/or adjacent oedema/haemorrhage) to grade 2 (partial interruption/thickening of the ligament and increased signal) and grade 3 (complete interruption–total rupture) to grade 4 (avulsion).[33,34]

Grade 1 changes at the origin and/or insertion of the ligaments are very common in joints with osteoarthritis (FIGURE 3D). Their clinical significance is questionable.

More severe ligament strain can lead to BELL changes at the origin or insertion; they may or may not be accompanied by grade 2 or grade 3 ligament changes.

Patella and Patellar Ligaments (Retinaculum and Ligamentum Rectum)

The patella and the ligamentum rectum are best evaluated on sagittal and transverse planes. The medial and lateral retinacula are best seen on the transverse plane, and the dorsal plane can help to verify a suspected lesion.

Apart from iatrogenic damage, rupture of the retinacula mainly occurs in cases with patellar luxation. In transient luxation, thickening or partial rupture of the retinacula can be the only signs of an unstable patellar position.

A "riding patella" is a rather common finding, which can occur due to the stifle position in an anesthetized dog; an extended position will lead to a relaxed patellar tendon and the patellofemoral joint will widen, allowing for mild patellar displacement. It should only be considered pathological in conjunction with signs of sprain injury of the patellar retinacula.

A partial rupture of the ligamentum rectum will lead to thickening and increased signal intensity of the ligament. In cases of total rupture, no ligament structure will be visible. The ligament is severely thickened and shows highly increased but usually inhomogeneous signal intensity.

Menisci

Whereas several sequences have been used in LF MRI to evaluate the menisci, the author prefers the GE T2*-w sequence for several reasons. It is available on all LF MRI scanners, provides excellent contrast between menisci and cartilage or joint fluid, is sensitive for pathologic changes and allows for high IPR and thin slices within a reasonable scan time. This sequence will show the normal meniscus as a slightly inhomogeneous hypointense, wedge-shaped structure with a smooth surface and sharp axial margins (FIGURE 4).

An alternative sequence would be the FSE PD weighted. It is not available on every machine on the market, and in many scanners the minimal slice thickness is restricted to 3 mm. High IPR can still be achieved, and it provides good contrast for evaluating meniscal lesions.The author recommends its use in the presence of metallic implants since it is less sensitive for field inhomogeneity artefacts than the GE T2*-w sequences (FIGURE 5).

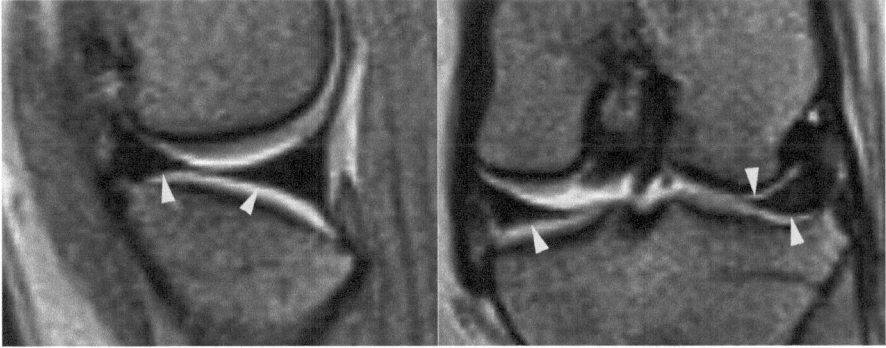

Figure 4. GE T2*-w images of the stifle of a normal 3 y M Newfoundland dog (69 kg). Sagittal (left; cranial is to the left) slice through the medial meniscus and dorsal image (lateral to the right) at the collateral ligament level demonstrating normal hypointense appearance of menisci (arrowheads). (VetMR, 0.19 T; Esaote, Genova, Italy)

In humans, several grading schemes for meniscal lesions exist.[35-39] In the veterinary literature, modified grading schemes or simple differentiation between tear and no tear have been used.[3,5,6,40,41]

As a general rule, it can be said that unsharp mild to moderate increase in signal intensity without contact with any meniscal surface is likely due to meniscal degeneration and is not clinically significant (FIGURE 3D). A sharply delineated linear increase in signal intensity without contact with any meniscal surface can be meniscal degeneration or an intrameniscal rupture. These grade 2 lesions do not seem to be clinically significant. As soon as the linear increased signal intensity is in contact with one or both meniscal surfaces, it

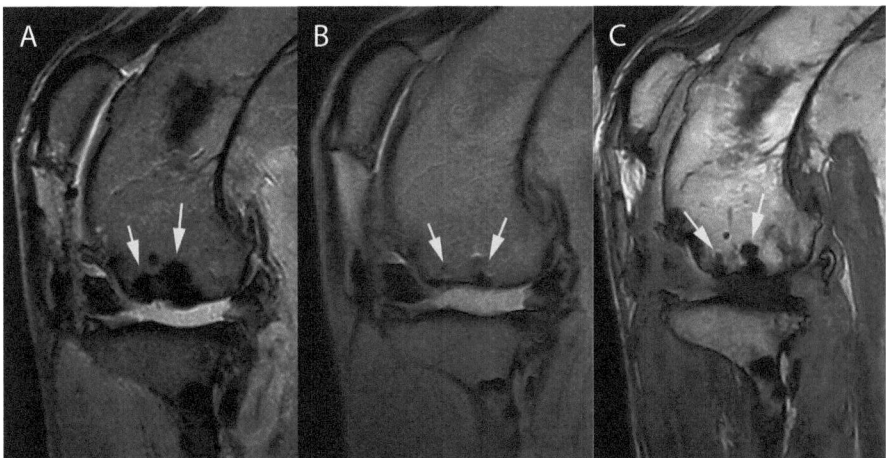

Figure 5. GE T2*-w (A), FSE PD (B) and 3D GE T1-w (C) sagittal images of the stifle of a 3 y M German Shepherd dog (35 kg). Images are oriented through the lateral femoral condyle in the presence of susceptibility artefacts due to previous surgery. The artefacts near the cartilage surface (arrows) are smallest in the FSE PD. (VetGrande, 0.25 T, Esaote, Genova, Italy)

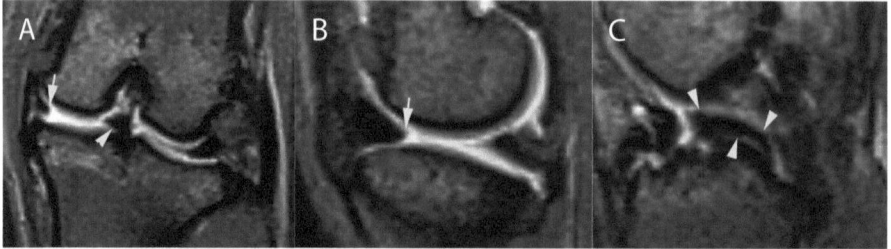

Figure 6. GE T2*-w images of the stifle of a 2 y F American Bulldog (37 kg) with a bucket handle tear of the medial meniscus. Dorsal (A, lateral is to the right) and sagittal images (cranial is to the left) through the medial femoral condyle (B) and the intercondylar area (C) are shown. (A) The axial border of the medial meniscus (short arrow) is blunted, and the axially displaced fragment (arrowhead) is visible. (B) A mildly blunted caudal border of the cranial horn (short arrow) is visible, and the axial part of the meniscal body is absent (compare to figure 4). (C) The displaced meniscal fragment is visible (arrowheads), sometimes appearing like a second caudal cruciate ligament. (VetMR, 0.19 T; Esaote, Genova, Italy)

is a meniscal tear and needs treatment. Deformation of the menisci with missing or displaced fragments are the result of complex and/or displaced tears and require treatment.

Axial meniscal fibrillation or fraying is not covered by most grading schemes,[35] most likely corresponding to axial fringe tears as described by Flo et al.[42] They can be recognized by slightly irregular or blunted axial margins in the absence of a displaced meniscal fragment (FIGURE 3B). Their clinical significance is still open but is most likely low, as long as they do not result in complete destruction of the meniscal body. Care must be taken not to confuse them with displaced longitudinal tears (bucket handle tear), where there will be a blunted axial border as well as an axially displaced fragment visible on dorsal plane images (FIGURE 6).

It is very important to carefully assess the meniscal contours in both planes to avoid missing meniscal tears. A tear running parallel to the slice orientation will not be visible if the orthogonal plane is not scanned (FIGURE 7). Any step or any discontinuity of a meniscal margin should raise suspicion of a tear.

A discoid meniscus, characterized by a disk-shaped meniscus covering the whole meniscal plateau, is a rare finding in dogs.[42,43] It can be considered an incidental finding but has to be differentiated from a bucket handle tear (FIGURE 8).

Cartilage

The LF MRI of cartilage remains a challenge. The cartilage layer thickness of the femorotibial joint ranges from 0.6 to 1.7 mm in dogs,[44,45] with the cartilage of the femoropatellar joint being even thinner.[46] In humans, cartilage MRI is

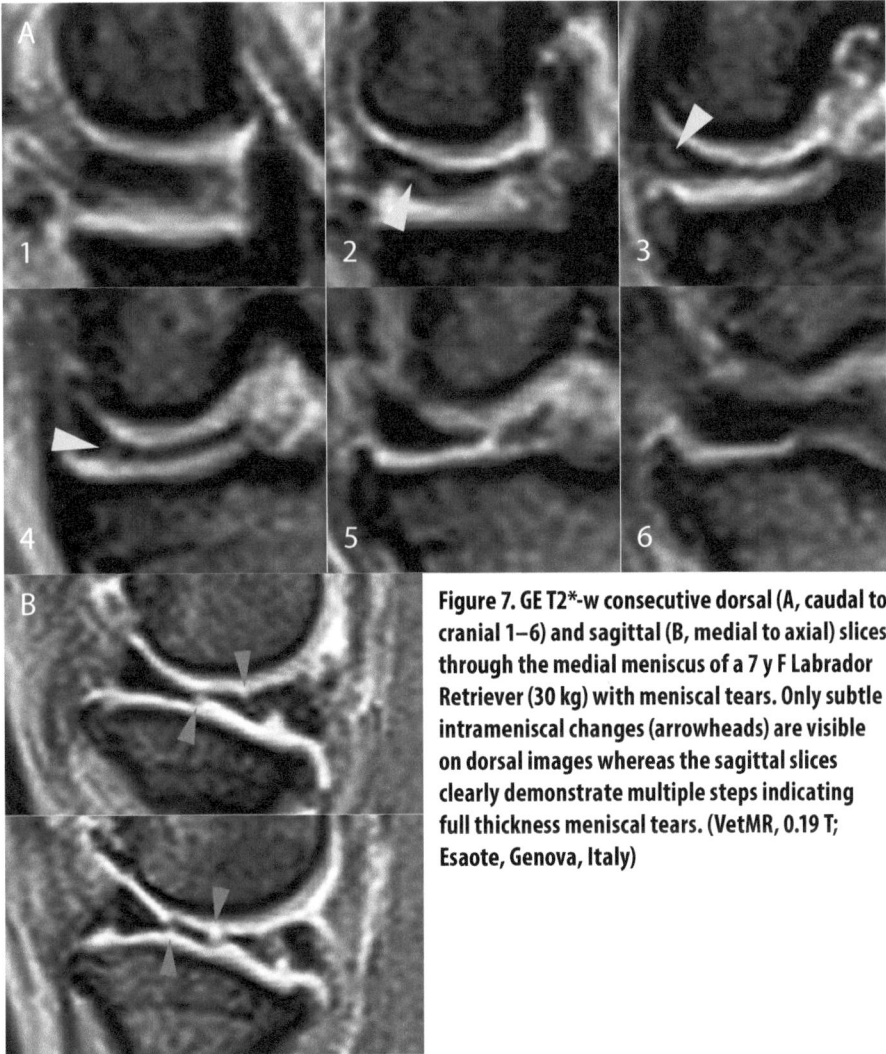

Figure 7. GE T2*-w consecutive dorsal (A, caudal to cranial 1–6) and sagittal (B, medial to axial) slices through the medial meniscus of a 7 y F Labrador Retriever (30 kg) with meniscal tears. Only subtle intrameniscal changes (arrowheads) are visible on dorsal images whereas the sagittal slices clearly demonstrate multiple steps indicating full thickness meniscal tears. (VetMR, 0.19 T; Esaote, Genova, Italy)

an area of intensive research and one of the reasons for the tendency to increase field strength.[47]

To the author's knowledge, the ability of LF MRI to visualize cartilage lesions in the canine stifle has not yet been evaluated. In a study correlating MRI findings of osteochondrosis lesions of the canine shoulder with arthrographic, arthroscopic and histologic findings,[48] cartilage was visualized on 5 mm thick slices, but the detection of loose cartilage flaps was unreliable. A more recent study faced difficulties visualizing the articular cartilage of the canine shoulder joint at LF MRI, but only spin echo sequences with 4 mm slice thickness were performed.[49]

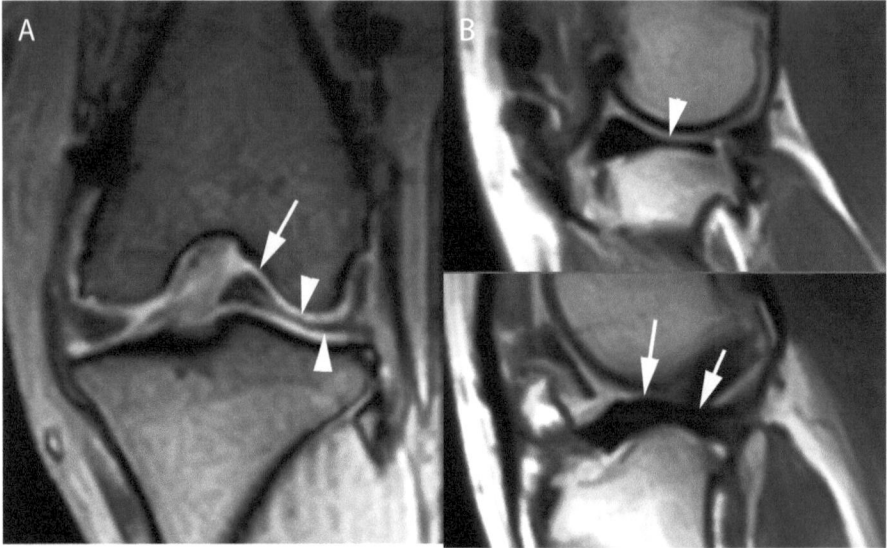

Figure 8. Images of the stifle of a 2 y F mixed breed dog (16 kg) with a discoid lateral meniscus. (A) Dorsal (lateral to the right) GE T2*-w at mid level of the intercondylar area shows broadened meniscal body (arrowheads) and thickened axial margin in the intercondylar area (arrow). (B) Sagittal FSE PD at mid level of the lateral femoral condyle and at the intercondylar area. The meniscal body is continuous (arrowhead), and the axial border is thickened and reaching far axially (arrows). (Aperto, 0.4 T; Hitachi Medical Systems, Düsseldorf, Germany).

Currently the only useful sequence for cartilage evaluation in LF MRI is a T1 weighted 3D GE (SPGR). It has been reported with different parameters for cartilage imaging in horses[50-52] and humans.[53] It allows high IPR (0.4 mm² @ 0.25 T, 0.9 mm² @ 0.2 T) and slice thicknesses between 0.7 and 1.1 mm. To evaluate the femoropatellar and femorotibial joints, it should be performed in sagittal orientation.

Normal cartilage will be shown as a mildly hyperintense (intermediate between fat and muscle) layer between the hypointense subchondral compacta and the hypointense joint fluid or menisci (FIGURE 9). The surface of the cartilage will be sharp and smooth, and the signal should be homogenous. Whereas larger surface defects can be detected easily (FIGURE 10), care must be taken in interpreting signal homogeneity and signal intensity of the cartilage. The 3D T1-w sequence is sensitive to inhomogeneity artefacts, magic angle effects and, especially in the smaller scanners (which need a smaller scan matrix), truncation and zero interpolation (ZIP) filling artefacts, which can mimic cartilage lesions (FIGURE 11). Subchondral oedema can be identified in STIR sequences and, to a slightly less reliable degree, with T1 weighting but may not be present underneath all cartilage defects. Intravenous contrast administration can lead to subchondral contrast uptake in more active lesions; however, it decreases cartilage contrast due to the generally increased signal intensity of enhancing background tissue (FIGURE 12).

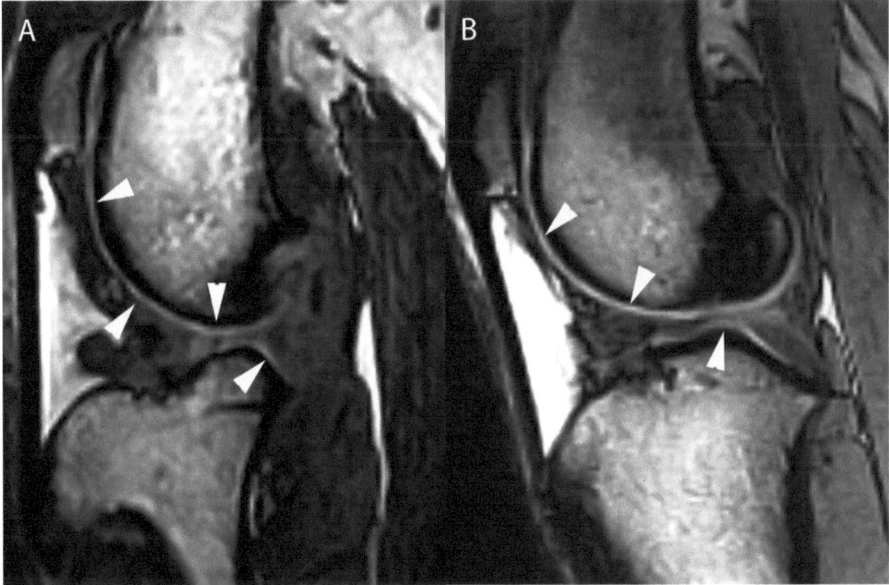

Figure 9. Sagittal 3D GE T1-w slices through the lateral femoral condyle demonstrating normal cartilage. (A) VetMR, 0.19 T, 7 y F Saupacker dog (46 kg); (B) VetGrande, 0.25 T, 4 y M Flat-Coated Retriever (50 kg); both Esaote, Genova, Italy. The cartilage can be seen as a bright line well delineated from the dark subchondral compacta (arrow heads).

Bone Marrow

The normal appearance of bone marrow on MRI changes with age.[54-56] The MRI appearance of the cartilaginous epiphysis and its transition to calcified bone containing red marrow in dogs has not yet been described. The youngest dogs with available MR images in veterinary literature were 4 months old. At that age the epiphysis already contains fat, resulting in high signal intensity in T1-w and low signal intensity in STIR images, whereas the metaphysis with red bone marrow has low signal intensity in T1-w and high signal intensity in STIR images.

The transition to adult (yellow) bone marrow appearance begins at 1 year and can last until the age of about 3 years. After that, normal bone marrow has high signal intensity in precontrast T1 weighted and low signal intensity in STIR sequences. However, bone marrow reconversion can occur for various reasons or just with age leading to signal distribution similar to that of young individuals.[54,57-59]

Focal increase in bone marrow signal on STIR images around the origin and insertion of the cruciate ligaments (BELLs) is a very common finding in joints with cruciate ligament disease.[32,60,61] Other focal changes of bone marrow signal include subchondral lesions in the case of cartilage defects, fractures

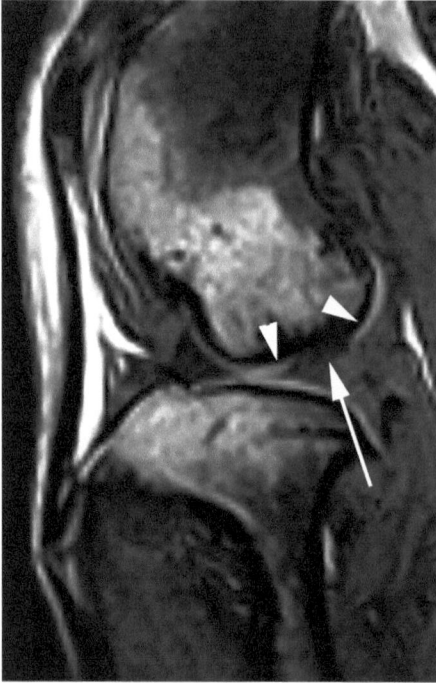

Figure 10. Sagittal 3D GE T1-w slices of a 4 y F German Shepherd dog (40 kg) with a cartilage defect. Images through the lateral femoral condyle demonstrate interruption (arrow) of the bright cartilage layer (arrowheads) indicating a full thickness cartilage defect. (VetMR, 0.19 T; Esaote, Genova, Italy)

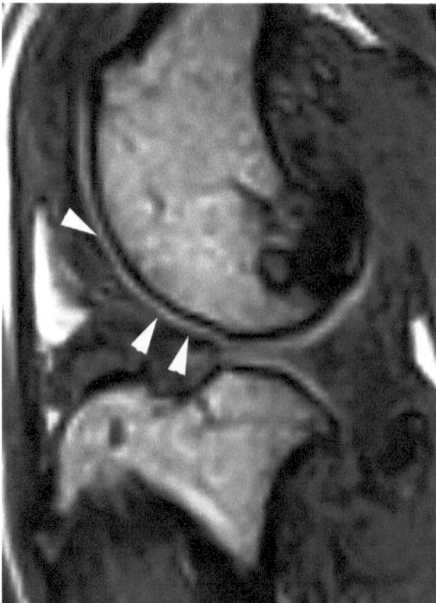

Figure 11. Sagittal 3D GE T1-w slice through the lateral femoral condyle of a 3 y F Labrador Retriever (27 kg). The dark lines interrupting the cartilage layer (arrowheads) are zero interpolation filling (ZIP) artefacts resulting from a mismatch between acquisition (192 x 160) and reconstruction (256 x 256) matrices. (VetMR, 0.19 T; Esaote, Genova, Italy)

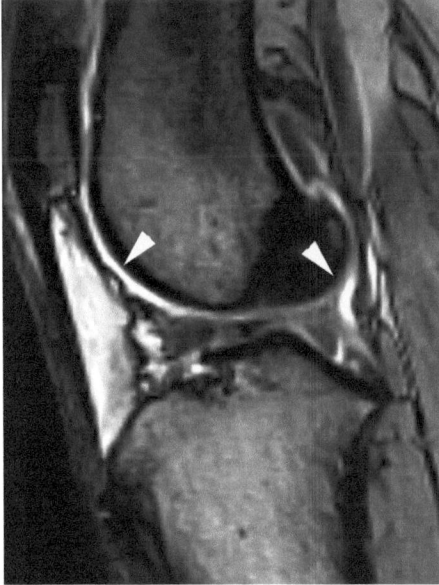

Figure 12. Sagittal contrast enhanced 3D GE T1-w slice through the lateral femoral condyle of a 4 y M Flat-Coated Retriever (50 kg). The visibility of the cartilage layer is reduced in comparison with the precontrast slice of the same dog in Figure 9B. (VetGrande, 0.25 T, Esaote, Genova, Italy)

and bone bruises (so called "footprint injuries", which indicate the direction and localisation of traumatic impact).[62-67]

Bone marrow metastases are focal or multifocal lesions, usually (but not always) bright on STIR and hypointense on T1-w sequences with contrast enhancement. Other than BELLs or subchondral bone lesions, they are not restricted to specific locations and are often round to oval.[68]

Diffusely infiltrating primary and secondary bone marrow disease can be difficult to detect since it results in diffuse and homogenous change of bone marrow signal.[69] It can be best seen on STIR images resulting in unusually bright bone marrow signal. On precontrast T1-w sequences, the changes are less obvious, showing diffuse and usually mild decrease of normal fat signal.

Extraarticular Structures

The best sequences for evaluating extraarticular structures are the STIR (a sagittal plane is preferable, but the dorsal plane of the standard protocol is an acceptable compromise) and the transverse T2-w sequences. Intravenous administration of contrast may be necessary to detect subtle strain injuries or partial rupture of the musculature. In these cases, pre- and postcontrast T1-w sequences (3D GE in sagittal plane recommended) are required.

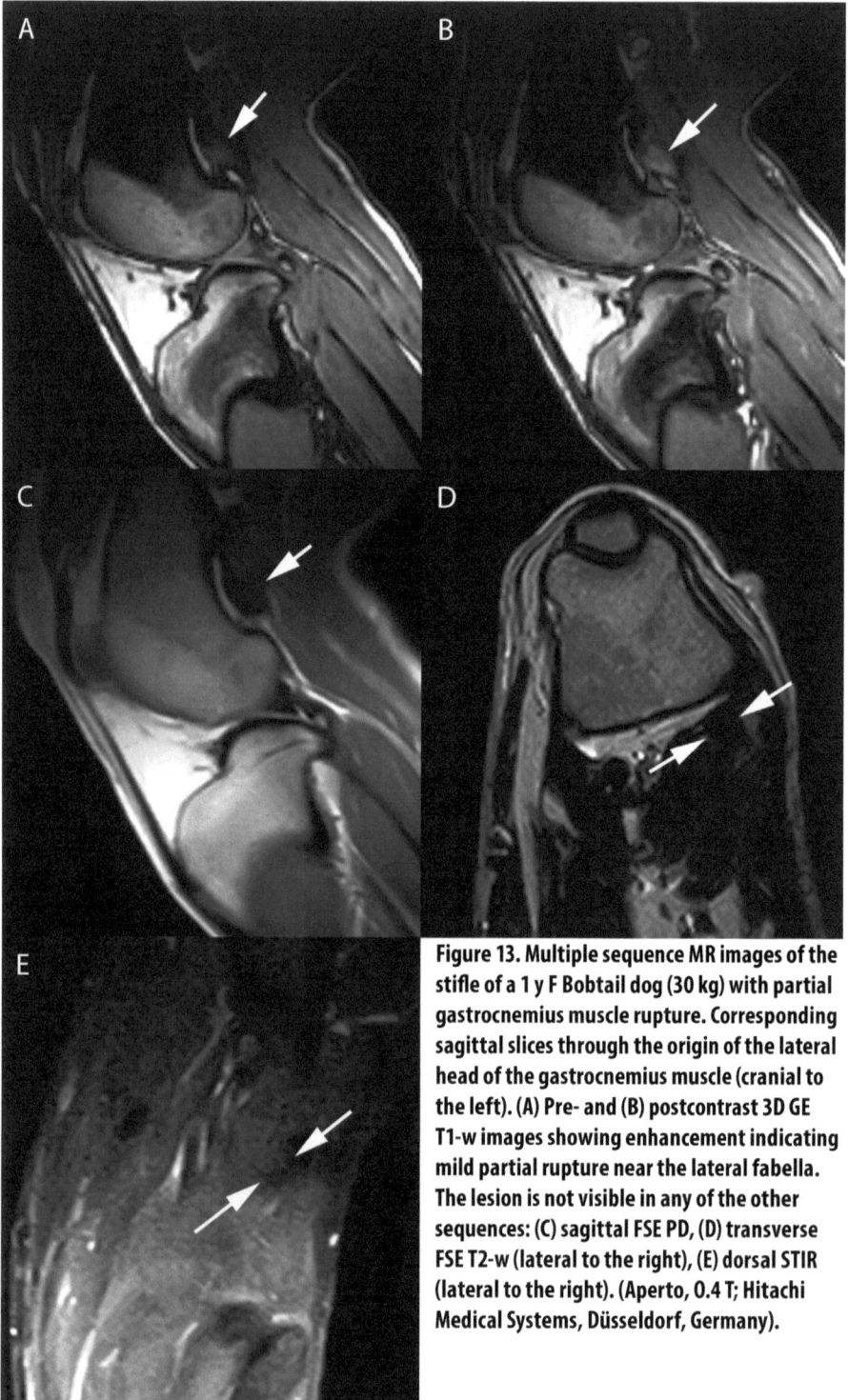

Figure 13. Multiple sequence MR images of the stifle of a 1 y F Bobtail dog (30 kg) with partial gastrocnemius muscle rupture. Corresponding sagittal slices through the origin of the lateral head of the gastrocnemius muscle (cranial to the left). (A) Pre- and (B) postcontrast 3D GE T1-w images showing enhancement indicating mild partial rupture near the lateral fabella. The lesion is not visible in any of the other sequences: (C) sagittal FSE PD, (D) transverse FSE T2-w (lateral to the right), (E) dorsal STIR (lateral to the right). (Aperto, 0.4 T; Hitachi Medical Systems, Düsseldorf, Germany).

Muscles

Partial ruptures of the proximal gastrocnemius muscle are rather common in herding dogs and their MRI appearance has been described,[70,71] but they can also occur in cats.

Diagnosis is straightforward; affected muscle areas show diffuse bright signal intensity in fluid sensitive sequences, usually around or shortly distal to the fabellae. In subtle cases, the lesions can be invisible on precontrast sequences, and contrast is necessary to detect them (FIGURE 13).

In cases of severe partial or total rupture, the affected muscle part can show a target like appearance on transverse FSE T2-w sequences. The hypointense separated fibres or tendon in the centre are surrounded by a circular hyperintense area of fluid accumulation that mimics the appearance of a tendon sheath.

Avulsions of muscle tendons result in a bony defect at the origin/insertion of the tendon, often surrounded by a sclerotic margin that is hypointense in all sequences. It becomes impossible to follow the tendon along its normal course, and the separated muscle will again be surrounded by fluid and/or haemorrhage.[72] Sometimes the bony fragment can be identified as a hypointense structure at the end of the separated tendon (FIGURE 14). In chronic cases, the avulsion bed and discontinuity of the tendon will still be present, but mainly hypointense fibrin or scar tissue replaces the fluid accumulation around the separated muscle.

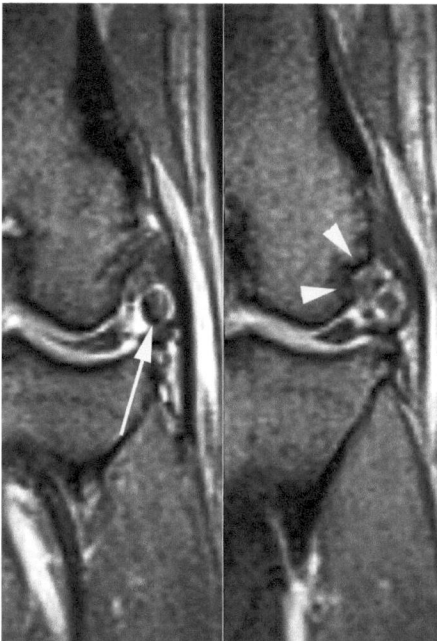

Figure 14. Consecutive dorsal GE T2*-w slices (lateral to the right) of the stifle of an 8 y M mixed breed dog (50 kg) with popliteus tendon avulsion. Images are oriented from caudal to cranial through the lateral femoral condyle. In the course of the popliteal tendon, there is a round bony fragment (arrow) visible. The avulsion bed at the tendon origin shows a bony defect with irregular margins (arrowheads). (VetMR, 0.19 T; Esaote, Genova, Italy)

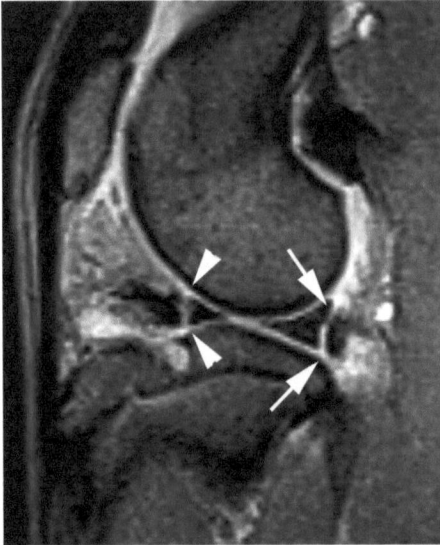

Figure 15. Sagittal GE T2*-w image of a 2 y M Labrador Retriever (37 kg) through the lateral femoral condyle (cranial to the left). The origin of the transverse ligament (arrowheads) and the popliteal tendon crossing the caudal horn of the lateral meniscus (arrows) mimic vertical meniscal ruptures. (VetMR, 0.19 T; Esaote, Genova, Italy)

Lymph Nodes

The popliteal lymph node is normally ovoid, sharply delineated and isointense to muscle in T2-w and precontrast T1-w sequences and hyperintense on STIR sequences. The normal lymph node enhances after intravenous contrast administration.

A common finding is a reactive lymph node with mild to moderate enlargement and increased signal intensity in T2-w images (up to isointensity with fluid). Contrast uptake is normal or increased. Lack of contrast uptake in an enlarged lymph node is a bad sign that should prompt fine needle aspiration (FNA) and/or biopsy. The author has seen this only with neoplastic infiltration.

The Post Surgical Stifle

The main concern in LF MRI of previously operated stifle joints is with artefacts arising from surgical implants, suture material and debris of drilling devices.[6,73,74] The size and localisation of the metallic disturbances and their impact on the diagnostic quality of the study depend on the material of the implant, its size, its orientation in relation to the magnetic field and its position. In HF MRI, common implants cause local artefacts but will usually still allow evaluation of intraarticular structures.[73,75] By choosing less susceptibility sensitive sequences (FSE, SE, GE, in order of preference) and adapting the scan parameters, such as swapping frequency/phase encoding direction, increasing readout bandwidth and reducing echo time, the artefact size can be reduced.[74] In the author's experience, in LF MRI even T2*-w GE sequences can still be used; an alternative is the FSE PD sequence. Unfortunately, the

3D GE T1-w sequence is also very susceptible to metal-related artefacts, and cartilage evaluation can become impossible in some cases (FIGURE 5).

Pseudolesions

Apart from technical artefacts, which can occur at every location in the body, the anatomy of the stifle joint provides several structures capable of mimicking lesions, especially of the menisci.

Ligamentum Transversum Genus

The ligamentum transversum genus connects the cranial horns of the menisci. At its origin it can easily mimic a vertical tear on sagittal images (FIGURE 15).

Popliteus Muscle Tendon

The intraarticular tendon crosses the caudal border of the lateral meniscus in an oblique plane. The caudal horn can seem ruptured, especially with a small amount of effusion in the tendon sheath (Figures 15, 16).

Extensor Digitorum Longus Muscle

The origin of this muscle is also surrounded by an intraarticular tendon sheath. This tendon sheath can lead to partial volume effects that mimic a meniscal lesion of the cranial third of the lateral meniscus (FIGURE 17A).

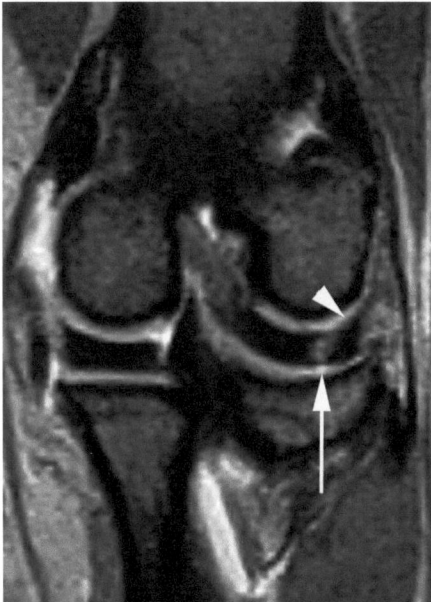

Figure 16. Dorsal GE T2*-w image of the stifle of a 2 y F Broholmer dog (49 kg) at the level of the caudal horns of the menisci (cranial to the left). The crossing of the popliteal tendon (arrowhead) can mimic a meniscal tear (arrow). (VetMR, 0.19 T; Esaote, Genova, Italy)

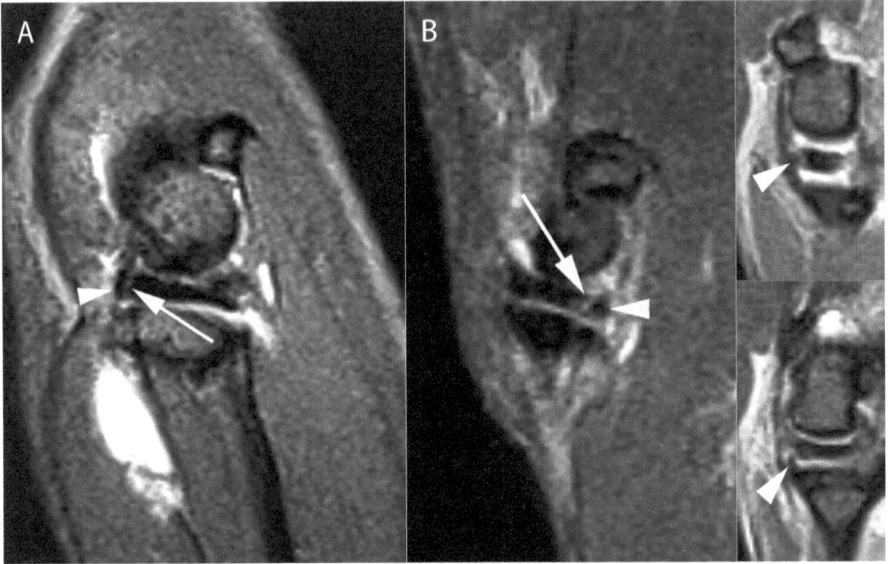

Figure 17. MR images of a 3 y F Labrador Retriever (27 kg) (A) and a 4 y F mixed breed dog (21 kg) (B) with M. extensor digitorum tendon (A, arrowhead) and M. semimembranosus tendon (B, arrowheads) mimicking meniscal tears (arrows). (A) Sagittal slice through the lateral meniscus. (B) Sagittal slice through the medial meniscus and consecutive dorsal scans demonstrating the course of the M. semimembranosus tendon. All images are GE T2*-w. (VetMR, 0.19 T; Esaote, Genova, Italy)

Semimembranosus Muscle Tendon

This tendon passes between the abaxial border of the medial meniscus and the medial collateral ligament. It can also give the false impression of a meniscal rupture (FIGURE 17B).

Caudal Meniscocapsular Attachment

Described in humans,[76-78] this connection between the caudal horn of the medial meniscus and the joint capsule has let to false positive diagnoses of a meniscal degeneration/rupture of the caudal meniscal horn. Flo et al.[42] have described stretching and attenuation of this structure in cases of cranial cruciate ligament deficient stifle joints.

Normal connective tissue shows the same signal intensity as the normal meniscus and cannot be delineated from the caudal horn, thus leading to an incorrect estimation of the true size of the meniscus. In some cases the ligament alone will have changed signal intensity allowing differentiation from the caudal horn. Partial and total meniscocapsular separation can occur and mimic a rupture of the caudal horn of the medial meniscus (Figure 18).

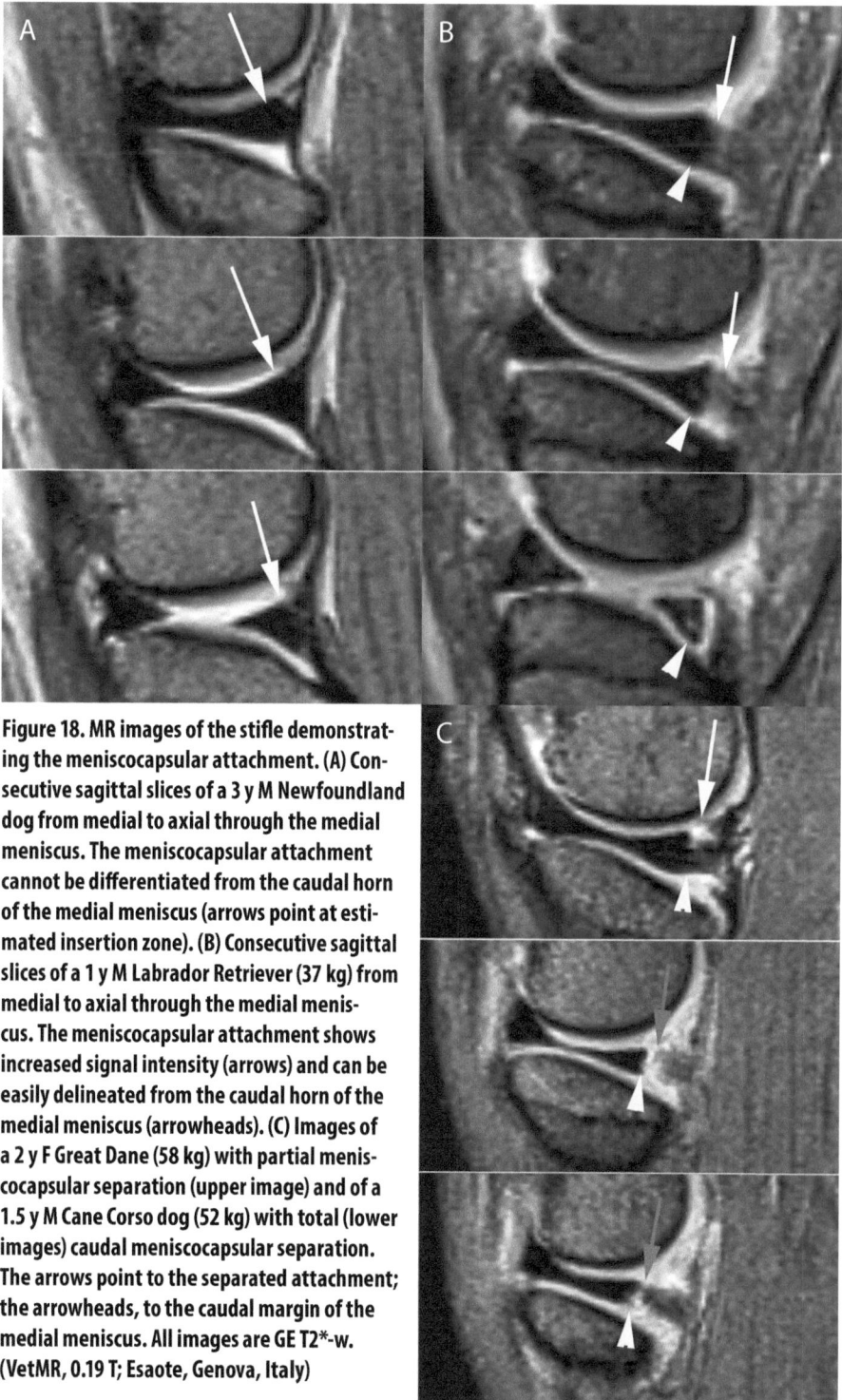

Figure 18. MR images of the stifle demonstrating the meniscocapsular attachment. (A) Consecutive sagittal slices of a 3 y M Newfoundland dog from medial to axial through the medial meniscus. The meniscocapsular attachment cannot be differentiated from the caudal horn of the medial meniscus (arrows point at estimated insertion zone). (B) Consecutive sagittal slices of a 1 y M Labrador Retriever (37 kg) from medial to axial through the medial meniscus. The meniscocapsular attachment shows increased signal intensity (arrows) and can be easily delineated from the caudal horn of the medial meniscus (arrowheads). (C) Images of a 2 y F Great Dane (58 kg) with partial meniscocapsular separation (upper image) and of a 1.5 y M Cane Corso dog (52 kg) with total (lower images) caudal meniscocapsular separation. The arrows point to the separated attachment; the arrowheads, to the caudal margin of the medial meniscus. All images are GE T2*-w. (VetMR, 0.19 T; Esaote, Genova, Italy)

Low-field MRI Is Still Promising for Imaging the Canine Stifle

Low-field MRI can provide high-resolution images with good contrast of the canine stifle joint. It just needs a little help. With optimized protocols and thorough knowledge of normal anatomy and variants, high diagnostic accuracy can be achieved.

Acknowledgements

The author wants to thank his clients for providing the image material used in this paper:

- Tierklinik Lüneburg, Lüneburg, Germany: VetMR, 0.19 T

- Ospedale Veterinario San Michele, Tavazzano con Villavesco, Italy: Vet-Grande, 0.25 T

- Tierklinik Haar, Haar, Germany: VetGrande, 0.25 T

- Tierklinik Hofheim, Hofheim am Taunus, Germany: Aperto, 0.4 T

References

1.   Baird DK, Hathcock JT, Kincaid SA, Rumph PF, Kammermann J, Widmer WR, et al. Low-field magnetic resonance imaging of early subchondral cyst-like lesions in induced cranial cruciate ligament deficient dogs. *Vet Radiol Ultrasoun.* 1998;**39**: 167-173.

2.   Baird DK, Hathcock JT, Rumph PF, Kincaid SA, Visco DM. Low-field magnetic resonance imaging of the canine stifle joint: normal anatomy. *Vet Radiol Ultrasoun.* 1998;**39**: 87-97.

3.   Bottcher P, Bruhschwein A, Winkels P, Werner H, Ludewig E, Grevel V, et al. Value of low-field magnetic resonance imaging in diagnosing meniscal tears in the canine stifle: a prospective study evaluating sensitivity and specificity in naturally occurring cranial cruciate ligament deficiency with arthroscopy as the gold standard. *Vet Surg.* 2010;**39**: 296-305.

4.   Gonzalo-Orden JM, Altonaga JR, Gonzalo-Cordero JM, Millan L, Orden MA. Magnetic resonance imaging in 50 dogs with stifle lameness. *Eur J Compan Anim Pract.* 2001;**11**: 115-118.

5.   Harper TA, Jones JC, Saunders GK, Daniel GB, Leroith T, Rossmeissl E. Sensitivity of low-field T2 images for detecting the presence and severity of histopathologic meniscal lesions in dogs. *Vet Radiol Ultrasoun.* 2011;**52**: 428-435.

6. Martig S, Konar M, Schmokel HG, Rytz U, Spreng D, Scheidegger J, et al. Low-field Mri and arthroscopy of meniscal lesions in ten dogs with experimentally induced cranial cruciate ligament insufficiency. *Vet Radiol Ultrasoun.* 2006;**47**: 515-522.

7. Bottcher P, Armbrust L, Blond L, Bruhschwein A, Gavin PR, Gielen I, et al. Effects of observer on the diagnostic accuracy of low-field MRI for detecting canine meniscal tears. *Vet Radiol Ultrasoun.* 2012;**53**: 628-635.

8. Stabler A, Glaser C, Reiser M. Musculoskeletal MR: knee. *Eur Radiol.* 2000;**10**: 230-241.

9. Steinbach LS, Palmer WE, Schweitzer ME. Special focus session. MR arthrography. *Radiographics.* 2002;**22**: 1223-1246.

10. Vahlensieck M, Peterfy CG, Wischer TK, Sommer T, Lang P, Schlippert U, et al. Indirect MR arthrography: optimization and clinical applications. *Radiology.* 1996;**200**: 249-254.

11. Coumas JM, Palmer WE. Knee arthrography. Evolution and current status. *Radiol Clin N Am.* 1998;**36**: 703-728.

12. Pujol E, Van Bree H, Cauzinille L, Poncet C, Gielen I, Bouvy B. Anatomic study of the canine stifle using low-field magnetic resonance imaging (MRI) and MRI arthrography. *Vet Surg.* 2011;**40**: 395-401.

13. Banfield CM, Morrison WB. Magnetic resonance arthrography of the canine stifle joint: technique and applications in eleven military dogs. *Vet Radiol Ultrasoun.* 2000;**41**: 200-213.

14. Wilke VL, Robinson DA, Evans RB, Rothschild MF, Conzemius MG. Estimate of the annual economic impact of treatment of cranial cruciate ligament injury in dogs in the United States. *J Am Vet Med Assoc.* 2005;**227**: 1604-1607.

15. Hayashi K, Manley PA, Muir P. Cranial cruciate ligament pathophysiology in dogs with cruciate disease: a review. *J Am Anim Hosp Assoc.* 2004;**40**: 385-390.

16. Ness M, Abercromby R, May C, Turner B, Carmichael S. A survey of orthopaedic conditions in small animal veterinary practice in Britain. *Vet Comp Orthopaed.* 1996;**9**: 6-15.

17. de Rooster H, de Bruin T, van Bree H. Morphologic and functional features of the canine cruciate ligaments. *Vet Surg.* 2006;**35**: 769-780.

18. Bennett D, Tennant B, Lewis DG, Baughan J, May C, Carter S. A reappraisal of anterior cruciate ligament disease in the dog. *J Small Anim Pract.* 1988;**29**: 275-297.

19. Knebel J, Meyer-Lindenberg A. [Aetiology, pathogenesis, diagnostics and therapy of cranial cruciate ligament rupture in dogs]. *Tierarztl Prax K H*. 2014;**42**: 36-47.

20. Johnson JM, Johnson AL. Cranial cruciate ligament rupture. Pathogenesis, diagnosis, and postoperative rehabilitation. *Vet Clin N Am-Small*. 1993;**23**: 717-733.

21. Harari J. Caudal cruciate ligament injury. *Vet Clin N Am-Small*. 1993;**23**: 821-829.

22. Jerram RM, Walker AM. Cranial cruciate ligament injury in the dog: pathophysiology, diagnosis and treatment. *New Zeal Vet J*. 2003;**51**: 149-158.

23. Johnson AL, Olmstead ML. Caudal cruciate ligament rupture. A retrospective analysis of 14 dogs. *Vet Surg*. 1987;**16**: 202-206.

24. Sumner JP, Markel MD, Muir P. Caudal cruciate ligament damage in dogs with cranial cruciate ligament rupture. *Vet Surg*. 2010;**39**: 936-941.

25. Comerford EJ, Smith K, Hayashi K. Update on the aetiopathogenesis of canine cranial cruciate ligament disease. *Vet Comp Orthopaed*. 2011;**24**: 91-98.

26. Podadera J, Gavin P, Saveraid T, Hall E, Chau J, Makara M. Effects of stifle flexion angle and scan plane on visibility of the normal canine cranial cruciate ligament using low-field magnetic resonance imaging. *Vet Radiol Ultrasoun*. 2014;**55**: 407-413.

27. Konar M, Kneissl S, Vidoni B, Lang J, Mayrhofer E. [Low-field MRI of the Canine Stifle Joint Part 1: Examination – Protocols and Sequences]. *Tierarztl Prax K H*. 2005;**33**: 5–14.

28. Reicher MA, Rauschning W, Gold RH, Bassett LW, Lufkin RB, Glen W, Jr. High-resolution magnetic resonance imaging of the knee joint: normal anatomy. *Am J Roentgenol*. 1985;**145**: 895-902.

29. Hodler J, Haghighi P, Trudell D, Resnick D. The cruciate ligaments of the knee: correlation between MR appearance and gross and histologic findings in cadaveric specimens. *Am J Roentgenol*. 1992;**159**: 357-360.

30. Baird DK, Hathcock JT, Rumph PF, Kincaid SA, Visco DM. Low-field magnetic resonance imaging of the canine stifle joint: Normal anatomy. *Vet Radiol Ultrasoun*. 1998;**39**: 87–97.

31. Zanetti M, Bruder E, Romero J, Hodler J. Bone marrow edema pattern in osteoarthritic knees: correlation between MR imaging and histologic findings. *Radiology*. 2000;**215**: 835-840.

32. Martig S, Boisclair J, Konar M, Spreng D, Lang J. MRI characteristics and histology of bone marrow lesions in dogs with experimentally induced osteoarthritis. *Vet Radiol Ultrasoun*. 2007;**48**: 105-112.

33. Newton CD, Farrow CS. Ligamentous Injury (Sprain). In: Newton CD, Nunamaker DM (eds): *Textbook of Small Animal Orthopaedics*. Philadelphia: Lippincott Company, 1985;843-851.

34. Stork A, Feller JF, Sanders TG, Tirman PF, Genant HK. Magnetic resonance imaging of the knee ligaments. *Semin Roentgenol*. 2000;**35**: 256-276.

35. Nguyen JC, De Smet AA, Graf BK, Rosas HG. MR imaging-based diagnosis and classification of meniscal tears. *Radiographics*. 2014;**34**: 981-999.

36. Firooznia H, Golimbu C, Rafii M. MR imaging of the menisci. Fundamentals of anatomy and pathology. *Magn Reson Imaging C*. 1994;**2**: 325-347.

37. Mesgarzadeh M, Moyer R, Leder DS, Revesz G, Russoniello A, Bonakdarpour A, et al. MR imaging of the knee: expanded classification and pitfalls to interpretation of meniscal tears. *Radiographics*. 1993;**13**: 489-500.

38. Crues JV, 3rd, Mink J, Levy TL, Lotysch M, Stoller DW. Meniscal tears of the knee: accuracy of MR imaging. *Radiology*. 1987;**164**: 445-448.

39. Stoller DW, Martin C, Crues JV, 3rd, Kaplan L, Mink JH. Meniscal tears: pathologic correlation with MR imaging. *Radiology*. 1987;**163**: 731-735.

40. Barrett E, Barr F, Owen M, Bradley K. A retrospective study of the MRI findings in 18 dogs with stifle injuries. *J Small Anim Pract*. 2009;**50**: 448-455.

41. Blond L, Thrall DE, Roe SC, Chailleux N, Robertson ID. Diagnostic accuracy of magnetic resonance imaging for meniscal tears in dogs affected with naturally occuring cranial cruciate ligament rupture. *Vet Radiol Ultrasoun*. 2008;**49**: 425-431.

42. Flo G, DeYoung D, Tvedten H, Johnson L. Classification of meniscal injuries in the canine stifle based upon gross pathological appearance. *J Amer Anim Hosp Assoc*. 1983;**19**: 325-334.

43. Ohlerth S, Lang J, Scheidegger J, Notzli H, Rytz U. Magnetic resonance imaging and arthroscopy of a discoid lateral meniscus in a dog. *Vet Comp Orthopaed*. 2001;**14**: 90-94.

44. Flatz KM, Glaser C, Flatz WH, Reiser MF, Matis U. [Detection and evaluation of cartilage defects in the canine stifle joint - an ex vivo study using high-field magnetic resonance imaging]. *Tierarztl Prax K H*. 2014;**42**: 291-296.

45. Frisbie DD, Cross MW, McIlwraith CW. A comparative study of articular cartilage thickness in the stifle of animal species used in human pre-clinical studies compared to articular cartilage thickness in the human knee. *Vet Comp Orthopaed*. 2006;**19**: 142-146.

46. Kiviranta I, Tammi M, Jurvelin J, Helminen HJ. Topographical variation of glycosaminoglycan content and cartilage thickness in canine knee (stifle) joint cartilage. Application of the microspectrophotometric method. *J Anat*. 1987;**150**: 265-276.

47. Recht M, Bobic V, Burstein D, Disler D, Gold G, Gray M, et al. Magnetic resonance imaging of articular cartilage. *Clin Orthop Relat R*. 2001: S379-396.

48. van Bree H, Degryse H, Van Ryssen B, Ramon F, Desmidt M. Pathologic correlations with magnetic resonance images of osteochondrosis lesions in canine shoulders. *J Am Vet Med Assoc*. 1993;**202**: 1099-1105.

49. De Rycke LM, Gielen IM, Dingemanse W, Kromhout K, van Bree H. Computed Tomographic and Low-Field Magnetic Resonance Arthrography: A Comparison of Techniques For Observing Intra-articular Structures of the Normal Canine Shoulder. *Vet Surg*. 2015.

50. Werpy NM, Ho CP, Pease AP, Kawcak CE. The effect of sequence selection and field strength on detection of osteochondral defects in the metacarpophalangeal joint. *Vet Radiol Ultrasoun*. 2011;**52**: 154-160.

51. Olive J. Distal interphalangeal articular cartilage assessment using low-field magnetic resonance imaging. *Vet Radiol Ultrasoun*. 2010;**51**: 259-266.

52. Santos MP, Gutierrez-Nibeyro SD, McKnight AL, Singh K. Gross and Histopathologic Correlation of Low-Field Magnetic Resonance Imaging Findings in the Stifle of Asymptomatic Horses. *Vet Radiol Ultrasoun*. 2015;**56**: 407-416

53. van der Linden E, Kroon HM, Doornbos J, Hermans J, Bloem JL. MR imaging of hyaline cartilage at 0.5 T: a quantitative and qualitative in vitro evaluation of three types of sequences. *Skeletal Radiol*. 1998;**27**: 297-305.

54. Konar M, Lang J. Age-related changes in MR Appearance of normal bone marrow in canine stifle joints. Abstract from the annual conference of the European association of veterinary diagnostic imaging. *Vet Radiol Ultrasoun*. 2004;**45**: 597.

55. Armbrust LJ, Hoskinson JJ, Biller DS, Wilkerson M. Low-field magnetic resonance imaging of bone marrow in the lumbar spine, pelvis, and femur in the adult dog. *Vet Radiol Ultrasoun*. 2004;**45**: 393-401.

56. Armbrust LJ, Ostmeyer M, McMurphy R. Magnetic resonance imaging of bone marrow in the pelvis and femur of young dogs. *Vet Radiol Ultrasoun*. 2008;**49**: 432-437.

57. Vande Berg BC, Malghem J, Lecouvet FE, Maldague B. Magnetic resonance imaging of normal bone marrow. *Eur Radiol*. 1998;**8**: 1327-1334.

58. Malkiewicz A, Dziedzic M. Bone marrow reconversion - imaging of physiological changes in bone marrow. *Pol J Radiol*. 2012;**77**: 45-50.

59. Andrews CL. From the RSNA Refresher Courses. Radiological Society of North America. Evaluation of the marrow space in the adult hip. *Radiographics*. 2000;**20**: S27-42.

60. Winegardner KR, Scrivani PV, Krotscheck U, Todhunter RJ. Magnetic resonance imaging of subarticular bone marrow lesions in dogs with stifle lameness. *Vet Radiol Ultrasoun*. 2007;**48**: 312-317.

61. Olive J, d'Anjou MA, Cabassu J, Chailleux N, Blond L. Fast presurgical magnetic resonance imaging of meniscal tears and concurrent subchondral bone marrow lesions. Study of dogs with naturally occurring cranial cruciate ligament rupture. *Vet Comp Orthopaed*. 2014;**27**: 1-7.

62. Schmohl M, Konar M, Tassani-Prell M, Rupp S. [Magnetic resonance imaging features of a caudal cruciate ligament rupture associated with a suspected bone bruise lesion in a dog]. *Tierarztl Prax K H*. 2014;**42**: 107-110.

63. Newberg AH, Wetzner SM. Bone bruises: their patterns and significance. *Semin Ultrasound CT*. 1994;**15**: 396-409.

64. Vincken PW, Ter Braak BP, van Erkel AR, Coerkamp EG, Mallens WM, Bloem JL. Clinical consequences of bone bruise around the knee. *Eur Radiol*. 2006;**16**: 97-107.

65. Vellet D. Magnetic resonance imaging of bone marrow and osteochondral injury. *Magn Reson Imaging C*. 1994;**2**: 413-423.

66. Cohen SB, Short CP, O'Hagan T, Wu HT, Morrison WB, Zoga AC. The effect of meniscal tears on cartilage loss of the knee: findings on serial MRIs. *The Physician Sportsmed*. 2012;**40**: 66-76.

67. Libicher M, Ivancic M, Hoffmann M, Wenz W. Early changes in experimental osteoarthritis using the Pond-Nuki dog model: technical procedure and initial results of in vivo MR imaging. *Eur Radiol*. 2005;**15**: 390-394.

68. Vanel D, Bittoun J, Tardivon A. MRI of bone metastases. *Eur Radiol*. 1998;**8**: 1345-1351.

69. Vande Berg BC, Lecouvet FE, Michaux L, Ferrant A, Maldague B, Malghem J. Magnetic resonance imaging of the bone marrow in hematological malignancies. *Eur Radiol*. 1998;**8**: 1335-1344.

70. Fiedler AM, Amort KH, Bokemeyer J, Kramer M. [Musculotendinopathy of the gastrocnemius muscle in a Labrador Retriever. A case report]. *Tierarztl Prax K H*. 2013;**41**: 349-354.

71. Stahl C, Wacker C, Weber U, Forterre F, Hecht P, Lang J, et al. MRI features of gastrocnemius musculotendinopathy in herding dogs. *Vet Radiol Ultrasoun*. 2010;**51**: 380-385.

72. Fitch RB, Wilson ER, Hathcock JT, Montgomery RD. Radiographic, computed tomographic and magnetic resonance imaging evaluation of a chronic long digital extensor tendon avulsion in a dog. *Vet Radiol Ultrasoun*. 1997;**38**: 177-181.

73. David FH, Grierson J, Lamb CR. Effects of surgical implants on high-field magnetic resonance images of the normal canine stifle. *Vet Radiol Ultrasoun.* 2012;**53**: 280-288.

74. Hargreaves BA, Worters PW, Pauly KB, Pauly JM, Koch KM, Gold GE. Metal-induced artifacts in MRI. *Am J Roentgenol.* 2011;**197**: 547-555.

75. Taylor-Brown F, Lamb CR, Tivers MS, Li A. Magnetic resonance imaging for detection of late meniscal tears in dogs following tibial tuberosity advancement for treatment of cranial cruciate ligament injury. *Vet Comp Orthopaed.* 2014;**27**: 141-146.

76. Kaplan PA, Gehl RH, Dussault RG, Anderson MW, Diduch DR. Bone contusions of the posterior lip of the medial tibial plateau (contrecoup injury) and associated internal derangements of the knee at MR imaging. *Radiology.* 1999;**211**: 747-753.

77. De Maeseneer M, Lenchik L, Starok M, Pedowitz R, Trudell D, Resnick D. Normal and abnormal medial meniscocapsular structures: MR imaging and sonography in cadavers. *Am J Roentgenol.* 1998;**171**: 969-976.

78. De Maeseneer M, Shahabpour M, Vanderdood K, Van Roy F, Osteaux M. Medial meniscocapsular separation: MR imaging criteria and diagnostic pitfalls. *Eur J Radiol.* 2002;**41**: 242-252.

6 SMALL INTESTINAL ULTRASONOGRAPHY IN DOGS AND CATS

Lorrie Gaschen[*] and Alexandre LeRoux[†]

[*]Louisiana State University, School of Veterinary Medicine, Baton Rouge, LA, USA

[†]Animal Medical Center, New York, NY, USA

The Importance of Ultrasonography in the Diagnosis of Small Intestinal Disease

Ultrasonography is a mainstay of diagnosing intestinal diseases in dogs and cats. This is partly due to its wide availability in general practice and its superior resolving ability. In dogs and cats with signs of gastrointestinal disease, ultrasonography combined with abdominal radiography is an important part of the minimum database. High-resolution (> 7.5 MHz) sonography allows the details of the intestinal wall to be assessed for layering, echogenicity and thickness, which are the main parameters used to diagnose intestinal wall disease.[1,2] Inappetence, anorexia, acute and chronic vomiting and diarrhoea and abdominal pain have numerous causes. Gastrointestinal ultrasonography is used extensively to help differentiate between inflammatory, infectious and neoplastic diseases, to rule out extraintestinal causes, such as pancreatitis and peritonitis, and to differentiate between functional and mechanical ileus when radiography is inconclusive. A major focus in veterinary medical research in the field of ultrasonographic imaging of the intestinal tract has been to discriminate between inflammatory, infectious and neoplastic disease. However, ultrasonographic assessment of wall layering is not always sufficient to identify intestinal pathology non-invasively.[1-6] Due to this, recent studies have described the use of additional descriptors such as layer echogenicity and relative wall thickness to diagnose and differentiate causes of intestinal disease. Ultimately, an equivocal result of the ultrasonographic examination

93

indicates the need for further diagnostic tests such as endoscopy and tissue sampling.

Although a negative test can be valuable in ruling out differential diagnoses, a recent study has challenged the usefulness of abdominal sonography in dogs with chronic diarrhoea when used as part of the minimum database.[7] That study assessed 87 dogs with chronic diarrhoea and found that in 66% of dogs, adding ultrasonography as part of the minimum database in the work up did not change the diagnosis. The conclusion was that ultrasonography was important in case management of chronic diarrhoea in 25% of dogs. A combination of chronic diarrhoea with weight loss, palpable abdominal or rectal mass, mixed bowel diarrhoea, older age category or persistent or constant diarrhoea were determined to be the best indications for the use of abdominal ultrasonography in those dogs. It should be noted that a majority of dogs in that study, however, had inflammatory or infectious disease, which according to established data, often presents with no or mild alterations to the intestinal wall. An important take home message is that the combination of chronic diarrhoea and a negative abdominal ultrasound should direct the clinician to the need for histopathological analysis.

Established Normal Ultrasonographic Parameters of the Small Intestine

The intestinal wall in dogs has five established alternating hyperechoic and hypoechoic intestinal layers: a hyperechoic lumen/mucosal surface, a hypoechoic mucosa, a hyperechoic submucosa, a hypoechoic muscularis propria, and a hyperechoic serosa.[6,8] No studies, however, have established direct comparisons between the thicknesses of the individual wall layers and histological layers, but the five-layer model is generally accepted (Figure 1). Relative wall layer thickness in healthy dogs and cats has also been established but not compared to histological measurements in the same animals.[9-11] Table 1 includes a list of references for small intestinal thickness in healthy dogs.

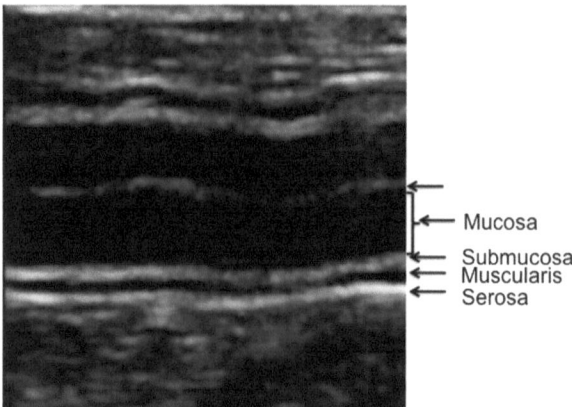

Figure 1. Longitudinal ultrasound image of a dog showing sonographic layering of the normal jejunum.

Mucosa
Submucosa
Muscularis
Serosa

Mean wall thickness in healthy dogs				
Author	Body weight (kg)	Layer	Jejunum (mm ± SD)	Duodenum (mm ± SD)
Delaney, et al.[8]	<10	total	3.22 ± 0.63	4.01 ± 0.77
	10-19.9	total	3.18 ± 0.64	4.00 ± 0.72
	20-29.9	total	3.33 ± 0.75	4.28 ± 0.70
	30-39.9	total	3.42 ± 0.70	4.52 ± 1.06
	>40	total	3.71 ± 0.74	4.56 ± 0.92
Stander, et al.[24]	2.3-5.0	total	2.5 ± 0.5	3.8 ± 0.5
Penninck, et al.[6]		total	2.25-3.0	
Gaschen, et al.[13]		total	3.3 ± 0.4	3.9 ± 0.5
Gladwin, et al.[11]	<15	total	3.0 ± 0.5	3.8 ± 0.5
		mucosa	1.8 ± 0.4	2.4 ± 0.5
		submucosa	0.5 ± 0.1	0.6 ± 0.1
		muscularis	0.5 ± 0.1	0.5 ± 0.1
		serosa	0.4 ± 0.1	0.4 ± 0.5
	15-30	total	3.5 ± 0.5	4.1 ± 0.7
		mucosa	2.0 ± 0.4	2.6 ± 0.6
		submucosa	0.6 ± 0.2	0.6 ± 0.2
		muscularis	0.5 ± 0.1	0.5 ± 0.1
		serosa	0.4 ± 0.1	0.4 ± 0.1
	>30	total	3.8 ± 0.4	4.4 ± 0.7
		mucosa	2.2 ± 0.5	2.8 ± 0.5
		submucosa	0.6 ± 0.1	0.6 ± 0.2
		muscularis	0.5 ± 0.2	0.6 ± 0.2
		serosa	0.4 ± 0.1	0.4 ± 0.1

Table 1. References for normal intestinal wall thickness and layering in dogs.

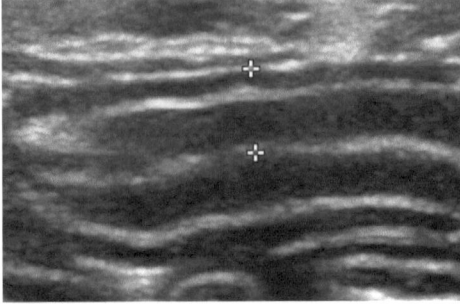

Figure 2. Longitudinal sonographic image of the jejunum in a 9-year-old cat with chronic diarrhoea for 5 years that was diagnosed with lymphocytic, plasmacytic and eosinophilic enteritis. The muscularis layer is thickened, but the wall has a normal total thickness of 3 mm.

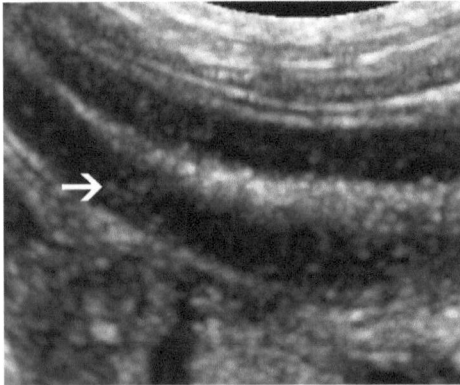

Figure 3. Longitudinal sonographic image of the duodenum in an 8-year-old female spayed Yorkshire terrier with confirmed inflammatory bowel disease and protein-losing enteropathy as well as hypoalbuminemia and a transudative peritoneal effusion. The cause of mucosal speckles (arrows) remains unclear.

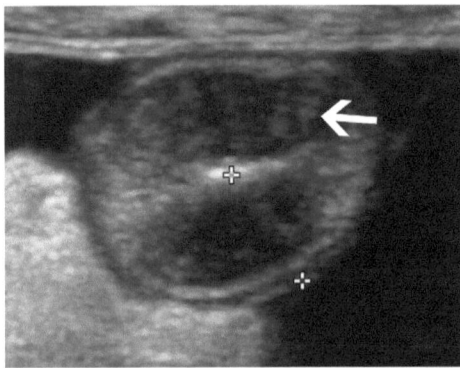

Figure 4. Transverse sonographic image of the jejunum in an 8-year-old female spayed Yorkshire terrier with confirmed inflammatory bowel disease and protein-losing enteropathy, hypoalbuminemia and a transudative peritoneal effusion. There are linear, hyperechoic striations (arrows) perpendicular to the long axis that represent lymphangiectasia.

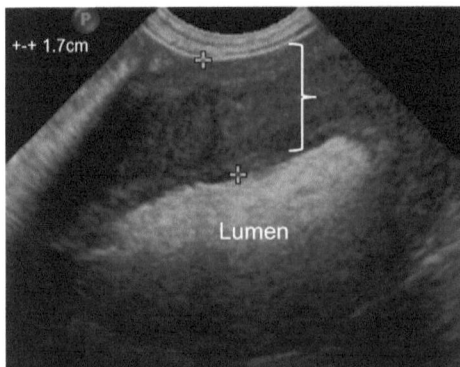

Figure 5. Transverse image of the jejunum in a 1.5-year-old male Rottweiler with chronic diarrhoea and weight loss caused by pythiosis. The intestinal wall is severely thickened (bracket is total wall thickness) and there is pseudolayering present with alternating indistinctly marginated bands of variable echogenicity.

Established Ultrasound Abnormalities of Chronic Inflammatory Diseases

Enteritis is generally diffuse with minimal wall thickening or alteration in wall layering (TABLE 2). It may lead to mild transmural thickening of the intestinal wall with preserved wall layering.[3-5,12] However, those same studies also showed that the intestinal wall may appear sonographically normal. In some instances the wall layering can be indistinct or completely lost if ulcerative enteritis, fibrosis, edema, hemorrhage and/or severe lymphoplasmacytic infiltration are present.[2]

The relative thickness of the layers may also change while the total wall thickness remains normal. Selective muscularis thickening can be due to idiopathic muscular hypertrophy of the smooth muscle layer of the intestine, and has been commonly observed in inflammatory conditions (FIGURE 2).[2] The echogenicity of the mucosa may be altered in both lymphangiectasia and lymphoplasmacytic enteritis.[3] Hyperechoic mucosal speckles and striations can be identified in inflammatory disease but are non-specific for the cause and severity (FIGURE 3).[13] Lymphangiectasia can occur in dogs with inflammatory bowel disease, as a primary idiopathic disorder or secondary to other infiltrative diseases, including neoplasia. The ultrasonographic diagnosis in dogs with protein losing enteropathy rests on the ability to demonstrate hyperechoic striations that are aligned parallel to one another and perpendicular to the long axis of the intestine in combination with hypoproteinemia and hypoalbuminemia in dogs with diarrhoea (FIGURE 4).

Mean intestinal wall thickness—Dogs with infectious and inflammatory diseases				
Author	Disease	Layer	Jejunum (mm ± SD)	Duodenum (mm ± SD)
Stander, et al.[24]	Parvoviral Infection		2.6 ± 0.5	3.5 ± 0.6
Gaschen, et al.[13]				
IBD	Inflammatory Bowel Disease	total	3.7 ± 0.9	3.9 ± 1
FRD	Food Responsive Diarrhoea	total	3.3 ± 0.5	4.2 ± 0.6
PLE	Protein Losing Enteropathy	total	3.9 ± 0.8	4.7 ± 1.2

Table 2. Intestinal wall thickness in dogs with infectious and inflammatory bowel disease

Established Ultrasound Abnormalities of Infectious Diseases

Infectious causes of intestinal wall infiltration have sonographic findings similar to neoplasia and are most commonly seen with fungal infections with pythium and histoplasma.[2] A focal mass with loss of wall layering is most commonly associated with neoplasia; however, fungal infections may cause similar lesions. Pythiosis and histoplasmosis can lead to intestinal wall thickening with pseudolayering, transmural loss of layering or a focal mass (FIGURE 5).[13] Pseudolayering is as alternating bands of hyper- and hypoechoic tissue within the intestinal wall that does not correspond to the normal wall layers. The distribution of fungal infection in the intestine can be focal or multifocal, but is usually not diffuse. Regional lymph nodes are often severely enlarged, rounded or irregularly shaped, and hypoechoic or heterogeneous. Intestinal histoplasmosis has been reported in the cat and can spread to the entire abdomen and lungs.[2] Abdominal ultrasound of both dogs and cats with intestinal histoplasmosis can show lymph node enlargement, thickening of the muscularis layer of the small bowel, focal thickening of the ileum with loss of layering and free peritoneal fluid. These abnormalities are sonographically similar to those of lymphoma and other neoplasms. Histology is required for differentiation between neoplastic and non-neoplastic masses of the intestines and lymph nodes.

Established Ultrasound Abnormalities of Neoplastic Diseases

In dogs, wall thickness of neoplastic infiltrative lesions is statistically greater than that of inflammatory disease (0.5-7.9 mm versus 0.2-2.9 mm, respectively).[4] When loss of wall layering is identified sonographically, there is a 50 times greater likelihood of a diagnosis of neoplasia versus inflammation.[4] Neoplastic masses may have concentric or eccentric wall thickening with loss of wall layering. Neoplastic infiltration of the small intestine is also statistically shown to be more likely focal than diffuse, which is more common in inflammatory disease.[4]

The most common intestinal wall tumors in dogs are carcinomas, lymphoma, leiomyoma and leiomyosarcoma.[14-17] In cats, the most common causes of neoplastic intestinal disease are lymphoma, mast cell tumor and adenocarcinomas. Visceral hemangiosarcoma involving the small intestine and colon has also been reported recently in cats, however, the sonographic characteristics have not been well established.[18]

There are no pathognomonic signs in dogs or cats for lymphoma.[19] In a recent study of nine dogs with small intestinal lymphoma, three had a sonographically normal wall thickness, two of them with normal layering and two with normal echogenicity.

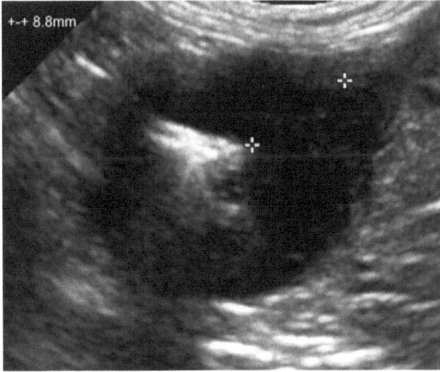

Figure 6. 16-year-old male neutered domestic long-haired cat with diarrhoea and weight loss caused by lymphoma. Transverse image of a jejunal segment affected by a focal lesion with severe wall thickening, transmural hypoechogenicity and loss of wall layering.

Alimentary lymphoma can be diffuse in both dogs and cats but most commonly occurs as a solitary, hypoechoic intestinal mass with transmural loss of wall layering (FIGURE 6).[2,14] Lymphoma is the most common neoplasm that causes diffuse infiltration and wall thickening that can appear similar to inflammatory disease (FIGURE 7). Thickening of the muscularis layer has been reported in inflammatory bowel disease and intestinal lymphoma in cats.[20,21] A recent study showed a significant association between muscularis thickening and feline T-cell lymphoma.[20] Cats in that study with lymphoma limited to the mucosa and lamina propria based on histopathology had no ultrasound abnormalities of the intestinal wall.

Due to the overlap of diseases associated with muscularis thickening and lymphadenopathy in cats, full thickness intestinal biopsies are likely indicated for a definitive diagnosis.

Intestinal adenocarcinoma in dogs and cats appears sonographically as transmural thickening with complete loss of wall layering.[2,14] This appearance is very similar to that of alimentary lymphoma when it forms a mass. However, carcinomas are usually solitary whereas lymphoma can be focal, multifocal or diffuse.

Intestinal smooth muscle tumors such as leiomyosarcomas often become very large and have an eccentric growth out of the intestinal wall through the serosa.[2] Leiomyomas tend to be small and appear as a focal intramural hypoechoic thickening with loss of wall layering. Intestinal mast cell tumors are less common and their appearance is similar to that of lymphoma as they cause hypoechoic transmural thickening of the wall with loss of layering.

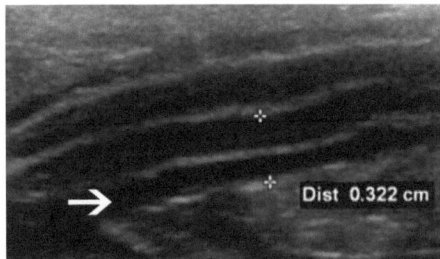

Figure 7. 13-year-old cat with a one-year history of watery diarrhoea caused by lymphoma. Sonographic images of the jejunum show diffuse muscularis thickening (arrow).

The majority of feline intestinal mast cell tumors are sonographically non-circumferential, with eccentric wall thickening, but can be asymmetric as well with a normal wall on the

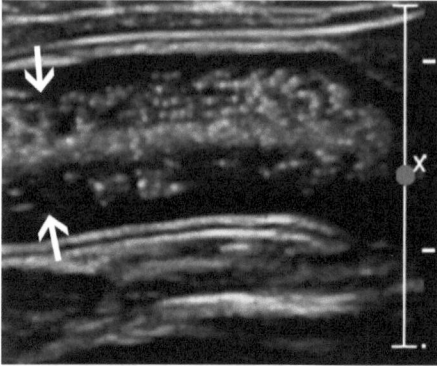

Figure 8. Longitudinal image of a canine duodenum 60 minutes after ingesting a meal mixed with corn oil. The intestinal mucosa has a hyperechoic mucosal border adjacent to the lumen (arrows).

opposite side.[22] These findings are in contrast to feline gastrointestinal lymphoma, which generally leads to circumferential symmetric transmural thickening of the intestine.

Latest Updates in Intestinal Ultrasonography

Mucosal Echogenicity

Mucosal speckles have been observed with intestinal inflammatory disease but their origin remains unclear. They may represent focal accumulation of reflective substances in the mucosal crypts (e.g., mucus, cellular debris, protein, mineralized or fibrous tissue, or gas).[13,23-25] A recent study examined the effects of oral corn oil administration and the presence of mucosal striations in healthy small breed dogs and those with histopathologically diagnosed lymphangiectasia.[26] It was established that mucosal striations in the duodenum and jejunum in dogs with histopathologically confirmed lymphangiectasia were usually present prior to corn oil administration but their visualization was enhanced with corn oil at 60 and 90 minutes post-prandial.[26] Only one control dog in that study developed mucosal striations after corn oil administration but 4/5 developed increased echogenicity, mainly due to speckles, as early as 30 minutes post corn oil administration (FIGURE 8). However, the effect of a recent regular meal on the mucosal echogenicity of the small intestinal mucosa has not been established in healthy dogs.

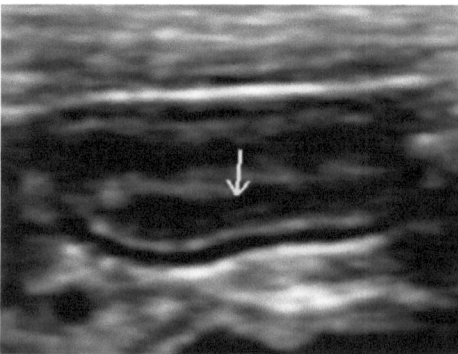

Figure 9. 12-year-old domestic short hair cat with chronic renal disease. A thin hyperechoic line is present within the mucosal layer (arrow). The hyperechoic line was diffuse throughout the mucosa and its cause was unknown.

In a study of 11 cats,[27] a hyperechoic line within the mucosa parallel to the submucosa has been correlated histologically with small intestinal mucosal fibrosis. In that study,[27] it was mainly observed within the jejunum compared to the duodenum, but was not reported in the ileum of any of the 11 cats included (FIGURE 9). A similar echogenic mucosal line has also been reported more recently in dogs.[26] In this recent study, following oral administration of corn

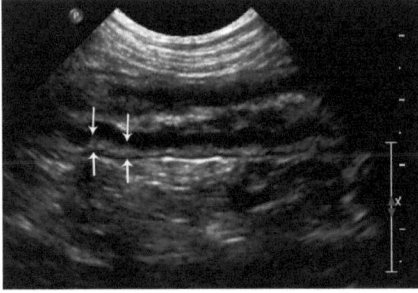

Figure 10. Longitudinal ultrasound image of the jejunum of a dog diagnosed with schistosomiasis due to Heterobilharzia americanum. The longitudinal jejunal segment shows a thickened, indistinctly marginated hyperechoic submucosal layer (arrow).

oil, a mucosal hyperechoic line running parallel to the submucosa became visible in the duodenum and jejunum of healthy dogs and dogs diagnosed with lymphangiectasia and was assumed to represent a dilated lymphatic vessel, responsible for uptake of fat from the lacteals, becoming more conspicuous after corn oil administration because of its distension.[26] However, despite the transient feature of this ultrasound finding, which made a lymphatic dilation a possible source, this assumption was not confirmed histologically. At this time, the clinical significance of a hyperechoic line in the mucosa, parallel to the submucosa, is of unknown clinical significance.

Submucosal Layer

Abnormalities isolated to the submucosal layer of the small intestinal wall are not common. Recently, thickening of the submucosa has been identified with *Heterobilharzia americana* infection. *H. americana* is a liver fluke whose natural definitive host includes raccoons and nutria but the domestic dog is susceptible to infection which is referred to as schistosomiasis.[28] Sonographically, the submucosal layer may be thickened and indistinctly marginated (FIGURE 10).[28] Both the gastric and small intestinal wall can be affected and if dystrophic mineralization is present, twinkling artifact with color Doppler may be detected.

Muscularis Layer

Recently, relative layer thicknesses of the cat have been reported and the muscularis layer of healthy cats was statistically significantly greater than half the thickness of the submucosa.[9] This is important as an earlier work defined an abnormal muscularis layer as being greater than half the thickness of the submucosa.[20] This was not the case, however, in a similar study that showed the two layers to be similar in thickness in healthy cats (TABLE 3).[10] The authors of the original work describing muscularis thickening in cats with T-cell lymphoma have now recently reported in a new follow-up study that there is a significantly increased thickness of the muscularis propria in cats with lymphoma and inflammatory bowel disease compared with healthy cats.[29] The mean thickness of the muscularis propria in cats with lymphoma or inflammatory bowel disease in that study was twice the thickness of that of healthy cats, and was the major contributor to significant overall bowel wall thickening in the

Mean intestinal wall thickness in healthy cats			
Author	**Layer**	**Jejunum** (mm ± SD)	**Duodenum** (mm ± SD)
Penninck, et al.[10]	total	2.22 ± 0.18	2.20 ± 0.17
	mucosa	1.20 ± 0.14	1.27 ± 0.15
	submucosa	0.36 ± 0.04	0.36 ± 0.04
	muscularis	0.35 ± 0.05	0.28 ± 0.07
Winter, et al.[9]	total	2.3	2.4
	mucosa	1.1	1.4
	submucosa	0.3	0.3
	muscularis	0.4	0.4

Table 3. Intestinal wall thickness in healthy cats

duodenum and jejunum. This new study established a muscularis to submucosa ratio >1 to be indicative of an abnormal bowel segment. The take home message of these new studies is that a thickened muscularis layer in cats can be found in either lymphoma or inflammatory disease and histopathology is still necessary to establish a diagnosis.

References

1. Penninck D. Gastrointestinal tract. In: Nyland, TG, Mattoon, JS(eds): *Small Animal Diagnostic Ultrasound*: Saunders, 2002;207-230.

2. Penninck D. Gastrointestinal tract In: Penninck, D, d'Anjou, M-A(eds): *Atlas of small animal ultrasonography*. Ames, Iowa: Blackwell Pub., 2008;281-318.

3. Gaschen L. Ultrasonography of small intestinal inflammatory and neoplastic diseases in dogs and cats. *Vet Clin North Am Small Anim Pract*. 2011;**41**:329-344.

4. Larson MM, Biller DS. Ultrasound of the gastrointestinal tract. *Vet Clin North Am Small Anim Pract*. 2009;**39**:747-759.

5. Penninck D, Smyers B, Webster CR, Rand W, Moore AS. Diagnostic value of ultrasonography in differentiating enteritis from intestinal neoplasia in dogs. *Vet Radiol Ultrasound*. 2003;**44**:570-575.

6. Penninck DG, Nyland TG, Fisher PE, Kerr LY. Ultrasonography of the normal canine gastrointestinal tract. *Vet Radiol*. 1989;**30**:272-276.

7. Leib MS, Larson MM, Grant DC, Monroe WE, Troy GC, Panciera DL, et al. Diagnostic utility of abdominal ultrasonography in dogs with chronic diarrhea. *J Vet Intern Med.* 2012;**26**:1288-1294.

8. Delaney F, O'Brien RT, Waller K. Ultrasound evaluation of small bowel thickness compared to weight in normal dogs. *Vet Radiol Ultrasound.* 2003;**44**:577-580.

9. Winter MD, Londono L, Berry CR, Hernandez JA. Ultrasonographic evaluation of relative gastrointestinal layer thickness in cats without clinical evidence of gastrointestinal tract disease. *J Feline Med Surg.* 2014;**16**:118-124.

10. Di Donato P, Penninck D, Pietra M, Cipone M, Diana A. Ultrasonographic measurement of the relative thickness of intestinal wall layers in clinically healthy cats. *J Feline Med Surg.* 2014;**16**:333-339.

11. Gladwin NE, Penninck DG, Webster CR. Ultrasonographic evaluation of the thickness of the wall layers in the intestinal tract of dogs. *Am J Vet Res.* 2014;**75**:349-353.

12. Rudorf H, van Schaik G, O'Brien RT, Brown PJ, Barr FJ, Hall EJ. Ultrasonographic evaluation of the thickness of the small intestinal wall in dogs with inflammatory bowel disease. *J Small Anim Pract.* 2005;**46**:322-326.

13. Gaschen L, Kircher P, Stussi A, Allenspach K, Gaschen F, Doherr M, et al. Comparison of ultrasonographic findings with clinical activity index (CIBDAI) and diagnosis in dogs with chronic enteropathies. *Vet Radiol Ultrasound.* 2008;**49**:56-64.

14. Penninck DG. Characterization of gastrointestinal tumors. *Vet Clin North Am Small Anim Pract.* 1998;**28**:777-797.

15. Paoloni MC, Penninck DG, Moore AS. Ultrasonographic and clinicopathologic findings in 21 dogs with intestinal adenocarcinoma. *Vet Radiol Ultrasound.* 2002;**43**:562-567.

16. Monteiro CB, O'Brien RT. A retrospective study on the sonographic findings of abdominal carcinomatosis in 14 cats. *Vet Radiol Ultrasound.* 2004;**45**:559-564.

17. Yam PS, Johnson VS, Martineau HM, Dickie A, Sullivan M. Multicentric lymphoma with intestinal involvement in a dog. *Vet Radiol Ultrasound.* 2002;**43**:138-143.

18. Culp WT, Drobatz KJ, Glassman MM, Baez JL, Aronson LR. Feline visceral hemangiosarcoma. *J Vet Intern Med.* 2008;**22**:148-152.

19. Frances M, Lane AE, Lenard ZM. Sonographic features of gastrointestinal lymphoma in 15 dogs. *J Small Anim Pract.* 2013;**54**:468-474.

20. Zwingenberger AL, Marks SL, Baker TW, Moore PF. Ultrasonographic evaluation of the muscularis propria in cats with diffuse small intestinal lymphoma or inflammatory bowel disease. *J Vet Intern Med.* 2010;**24**:289-292.

21. Evans SE, Bonczynski JJ, Broussard JD, Han E, Baer KE. Comparison of endoscopic and full-thickness biopsy specimens for diagnosis of inflammatory bowel disease and alimentary tract lymphoma in cats. *J Am Vet Med Assoc.* 2006;**229**:1447-1450.

22. Laurenson MP, Skorupski KA, Moore PF, Zwingenberger AL. Ultrasonography of intestinal mast cell tumors in the cat. *Vet Radiol Ultrasound.* 2011;**52**:330-334.

23. Rault DN, Besso JG, Boulouha L, Begon D, Ruel Y. Significance of a common extended mucosal interface observed in transverse small intestine sonograms. *Vet Radiol Ultrasound.* 2004;**45**:177-179.

24. Stander N, Wagner WM, Goddard A, Kirberger RM. Ultrasonographic appearance of canine parvoviral enteritis in puppies. *Vet Radiol Ultrasound.* 2010;**51**:69-74.

25. Sutherland-Smith J, Penninck DG, Keating JH, Webster CR. Ultrasonographic intestinal hyperechoic mucosal striations in dogs are associated with lacteal dilation. *Vet Radiol Ultrasound.* 2007;**48**:51-57.

26. Pollard RE, Johnson EG, Pesavento PA, Baker TW, Cannon AB, Kass PH, et al. Effects of corn oil administered orally on conspicuity of ultrasonographic small intestinal lesions in dogs with lymphangiectasia. *Vet Radiol Ultrasound.* 2013;**54**:390-397.

27. Penninck DG, Webster CR, Keating JH. The sonographic appearance of intestinal mucosal fibrosis in cats. *Vet Radiol Ultrasound.* 2010;**51**:458-461.

28. Kvitko-White HL, Sayre RS, Corapi WV, Spaulding KA. Imaging diagnosis-heterobilharzia americana infection in a dog. *Vet Radiol Ultrasound.* 2011;**52**:538-541.

29. Daniaux LA, Laurenson MP, Marks SL, Moore PF, Taylor SL, Chen RX, et al. Ultrasonographic thickening of the muscularis propria in feline small intestinal small cell T-cell lymphoma and inflammatory bowel disease. *J Feline Med Surg.* 2014;**16**:89-98.

7 ABSTRACTS FROM GERMAN PUBLICATIONS 2014 AND EARLY 2015

Reprint of selected abstracts of work published in the Pferdeheilkunde in 2014-2015 with permission of the publisher. All abstracts and information on how to obtain full text articles are available on www.biblioserver.com/pferde-heilkunde-fundus/index.php.

Abstracts selected and edited by Sandra Martig

Centre for Animal Referral and Emergency (CARE), Collingwood, Victoria, Australia.

Radiological Findings in the Thoracic Spine of the Horse According to the German Radiographic Guidelines 2007 Considering the Clinical Relevance

C.P. Geiger & H. Gerhards. Pferdeheilkunde 2015; 31(1): 39-48.

Both veterinary surgeons and horse owners are becoming increasingly concerned about the existence of actual or only inapparent back disorders in horses. Very often, tension in the back, caused by painful limb disorders, or by inaccurate riding influence, for example, are misdiagnosed as diseases of the back. On the other hand, horses with severe radiological findings in the spinous processes do not show any clinical abnormalities at all. The objective of this paper was to assess X-rays of the caudal thoracic and cranial lumbar spine (T10 – L1) in accordance with the German X-ray classification guidelines (Röntgenleitfaden, RöLf) 2007 and relate them to numerical values, clinical and species-specific considerations. For this purpose, X-rays were taken of the saddle position area (T10-L1) of 404 horses. Prior to this, a detailed clinical examination of the back of each animal was carried out. Similarly, the species-specific features (sex, race, type of use, performance problems, muscular development) and the numerical values (weight, height, age) were determined.

We found evidence that radiological findings on the spinous processes in the area of the saddle position can also occur in clinically healthy horses. Nevertheless, considerable changes, as classified in the X-ray class III-IV according to the German X-ray classification guidelines 2007, occur distinctly more often in horses showing clinical and performance abnormalities. Type of use, anatomy, age, weight and height do have a distinct influence on the incidence of radiological findings on the spinous process.

Comparison of Radiographic Changes of the Proximal Third Metacarpal and Metatarsal Bones in Horses with and Without Proximal Suspensory Desmitis

M. Trump, E. Siegenthaler, P.R. Kircher , A. Fürst, F. Theiss. Pferdeheilkunde 2014; 30(6): 671-676

Medical records of horses examined from 1994 to 2011 at the Equine Hospital, Vetsuisse Faculty, University of Zurich, because of proximal suspensory desmitis (PSD) were reviewed. Radiographic changes visible on dorsopalmar and dorsoplantar projections of the proximal third metacarpal / metatarsal bone (MCIII / MTIII) were analysed with respect to localisation, degree of increased radiopacity, length, width and pattern of radiopacity in relation to sex, age, breed, duration and degree of lameness and affected limb of the horses. Results were compared with those from sound control horses. Horses with PSD had increased radiopacity, which was significantly more prevalent medially than laterally in the forelimbs ($p < 0.05$) and more prevalent laterally than medially in the hindlimbs ($p < 0.05$). The width of the area of increased radiopacity was significantly greater in the forelimbs than in the hindlimbs ($p < 0.05$). The pattern of increased radiopacity was diffuse in 102 (85.7%) horses and multifocal in the remaining 17 (14.3%). 35.3% (n = 6) of multifocal changes were detected on one of the front limbs, whereas 74.7% (n = 11) were diagnosed on the hind limbs. Mildly increased diffuse radiopacity, with a distribution pattern comparable to cases with PSD was detected in 15 of 60 control horses. In comparison to control cases, the degree of increased diffuse radiopacity was significant more pronounced in horses with PSD ($p < 0.001$). The multifocal pattern of increased radiopacity could not be detected in any of the control horses. The results aid in the interpretation of radiographic changes seen in horses with PSD. Whereas a diffuse increased radiopacity of the proximal MCIII / MTIII needs to be interpreted with caution, as a mild degree may be seen in sound horses, the multifocal distribution pattern seems to be a unique feature of horses with PSD.

3-Tesla Magnetic Resonance Imaging of the Equine Brain in Healthy Horses – Potentials and Limitations

K. Stuckenschneider, M. Hellige, K. Feige, H. Gasse. Pferdeheilkunde 2014; 30(6): 657-670

For evaluating neurological diseases, magnetic resonance imaging (MRI) has been widely recommended as the method of choice in human medicine. It has been proposed as a valuable tool in clinical diagnostics and research projects in veterinary medicine as well. The aim of this study was to elaborate optimal settings appropriate for an examination of the equine brain in a 3-Tesla homograph within an adequate examination time and with related optimal image quality. A key issue was the evaluation of those neuro-anatomical structures (formations of grey and white matter included) which were always clearly recognisable and, as such, were useful orientation landmarks. Furthermore, the average sizes of selected structures were measured in the magnetic resonance images in transverse views. MRI of 11 healthy horses was performed under general anaesthesia. After the examination the horses were euthanised, their heads were fixated by perfusion, the brain was removed and cut either in transverse, dorsal or sagittal slices (approximately 4 mm thick). Photographic images of these slices corresponded to the magnetic resonance images in the equivalent planes. In the anatomical slices, all visible neurological structures (gyri, nuclei, and formations of white matter) were identified. In the corresponding magnetic resonance images, these structures were evaluated with regard to the image quality (intensity, delineation). Those best visible were proposed as landmarks for orientation. The evaluation of the image quality was performed using a score system. In general, the anatomical slices displayed more details compared to the magnetic resonance images. In the latter, large nuclei, e.g. nucleus caudatus, could always be identified with certainty, whereas small nuclei, like those of the thalamic region or of the area of the medulla oblongata, could not be identified. The relation between operational effort and benefit was discussed considering the parameters 'acquisition time' (and related duration of general anesthesia) and 'image quality' (which depended on the selection of sectional planes and matrix sizes, as displayed in the proposed protocols).

Development of the Cross Sectional Area of Flexor Tendons in the Metacarpal Region of 2-year-old Horses of Different Breeds

A. Köster, A. Lindner, H. Gerhards. Pferdeheilkunde 2014; 30(5): 541-550

This study examined the development of the CSA of the superficial and deep digital flexor tendon (SDFT and DDFT) and of the accessory ligament of the DDFT (AL-DDFT) in both forelimbs of six 2-year-old Thoroughbreds (TB), ten 2-year-old Standardbreds (SB), five 2-year-old Quarterhorses (QH) and ten 2-year-old German Warmblood Riding horses (WB) during one year with the hypothesis that it would be different among breeds. The initial CSA measurements were done in the yearling QH in November and thereafter in March, July and November of their 2-year-old season, and in the horses of all other breeds the measurements were in January, April, August and December of their 2-year-old year. The CSA was measured with ultrasound at four cm intervals, starting four cm distal from the distal border of the accessory carpal bone down to the metacarpophalangeal joint. The TB and SB were in race training, the WB were halter trained and the 2-year-old QH were schooled for western riding. For the SDFT, breed, CSA at specific distances distal to the distal border of the accessory carpal bone, ($p < 0.001$ both) and the interaction of breed and the CSA at specific distances distal to the distal border of the accessory carpal bone were significant ($p < 0.05$), but there was no significant difference between forelimbs ($p > 0.05$). The overall CSA from all measurements points was smallest in QH, largest in TB and WB, with SB having a CSA measurement between the other breeds. The overall CSA of SDFT in TB did not change during the observation period. However, in QH and WB there were significant decreases in the CSA, and these decreases varied between the CSA measured at specific distances distal to the distal border of the accessory carpal bone. In addition, in SB there were significant increases in the overall CSA measurement of the SDFT, followed by a decrease from August to December with CSA returning to initial values ($p < 0.05$ at least for all). For the DDFT too, breed, CSA at specific distances distal to the distal border of the accessory carpal bone, as well as the interaction of breed and the CSA at specific measurement points were significant ($p < 0.001$ all), but there was no significant difference between forelimbs ($p > 0.05$). The overall CSA from all specific distances distal to the distal border of the accessory carpal bone of DDFT was smaller in QH than in the horses of the other breeds studied ($p < 0.01$). There were no significant differences in the overall CSA among the TB, SB and WB. Few changes in the CSA of DDFT at the measurement points occurred during the observation period in QH and TB. In contrast, the SB CSA in both forelimbs decreased at 4 cm, 8 cm and 12 cm during the year of observation. However, CSA increased 20 cm and 24 cm distal to the distal border of the accessory carpal bone between January and August, returning to the initial levels thereafter ($p < 0.05$ at least for all). In WB, CSA of DDFT decreased continuously during the observation period at several measurement points in both forelimbs (p < 0.01 at least). For the AL-DDFT, CSA measurements were taken at 4 cm and 8 cm distal of the distal border of the accessory carpal bone only. The size of AL-DDFT CSA differed among breeds and specific distances distal to the distal border of the accessory carpal bone (p < 0.001 both). QH had the smallest overall CSA (p < 0.01 at least) while among the horses of the other breeds, the overall CSA did not differ (p > 0.05 among all). The QH also did not have any change in the CSA of AL-DDFT during the observation year at any specific distance distal to the distal border of the accessory carpal bone or between limbs (p > 0.05). In comparison, SB CSA of AL-DDFT increased at the 8 cm measuring point in the left forelimb between January and August and then decreased below the initial value by December (p < 0.01). There were no changes of CSA of AL-DDFT in the left forelimb of TB, while in the right forelimb CSA increased continuously at 4 cm and 8 cm distal to the distal border of the accessory carpal bone between January and August and then returned to the levels measured in January (p < 0.05). In WB CSA of AL-DDFT decreased continuously during the year of observation at all measurement points in both forelimbs (p < 0.01 at least). In conclusion, the development of the CSA of flexor tendons in 2-year-old horses varied markedly among breeds and during the year of observation. It remains to be proven whether the changes are due to genetics only or the management and especially the physical training of the horses played a role.

Use of Tissue Doppler Imaging in Horses – Exercise Stress Echocardiography with Tissue Doppler Imaging in Healthy Horses and Horses with Cardiac Disease

C. Hopster-Iversen, H. Gehlen, P. Stadler. Pferdeheilkunde 2014; 30(4): 444-454

The evaluation of performance capacity with exercise testing is of particular importance in horses with mild to moderate valvular regurgitation as a possible cause of exercise intolerance, and a detrimental cardiac function is often first detected after exercise. The aim of the study was the comparison of myocardial velocities evaluated with Tissue Doppler imaging in healthy horses and horses with a cardiac disease. 20 adult warmblood horses without cardiovascular diseases and 40 horses with valvular regurgitation or atrial fibrillation were examined. The examination included a clinical examination and standard electro- and echocardiographic examinations at rest. Additionally, the left ventricular septum (IVS) and the left ventricular free wall (LVW) were evaluated with tissue Doppler imaging at rest and after exercise. The peak systolic (S), early diastolic (E-Wave) and late diastolic (A-Wave) myocardial velocities were analysed with colour-coded Tissue Doppler and imaging (TVI) and with PW-tissue Doppler imaging respectively. Horses with atrial fibrillation (n = 15) showed an increase of systolic myocardial velocities at rest (TVI: IVS: control: -3.92±1.54 cm/s, AF: -6.66 ± 3.26 cm/s, $p < 0.0001$, LVW: control: 7.14 ± 1.18 cm/s, AF: 10.03 ± 3.10 cm/s, $p < 0.0001$) and after exercise (PW: IVS: control: -13.37 ± 3.84 cm/s, AF: -17.15 ± 3.93 cm/s, $p < 0.005$, LVW: control: 13.53 ± 3.66 cm/s, AF: 17.95 ± 3.50 cm/s, $p < 0.001$) compared to the healthy control horses. Furthermore, the group of horses with atrial fibrillation had higher early diastolic myocardial velocities then the control horses (TVI: IVS: control: 12.34 ± 2.91 cm/s, AF: 16.70 ± 6.13 cm/s, $p < 0.001$, LVW: control: -17.32 ± 5.25 cm/s, AF: -22.25 ± 5.19 cm/s, $p < 0.01$). Horses with mitral valve regurgitation (n = 15) also had higher systolic myocardial velocities, but only at rest compared to the healthy control horses (PW: IVS: control: -8.36 ± 1.78 cm/s, MVI: -10.99 ± 3.13 cm/s, $p < 0.005$), while horses with aortic valve regurgitations (n = 10) had higher early diastolic myocardial velocities at rest (PW: IVS: control: 17.06 ± 3.85 cm/s, AVI: 20.30 ± 3.59 cm/s, $p < 0.05$), but higher late diastolic velocities after exercise compared to the healthy control horses (TVI: LVW: control: -8.62 ± 3.7 cm/s, AVI: -11.86 ± 2.05 cm/s, $p < 0.05$). The myocardial analysis with tissue Doppler imaging was feasible at rest and after exercise. The increase of myocardial velocities in the horses with cardiovascular disease is probably the result of an increase in contractility due to increased filling pressure of the ventricle in the presence of adequate ventricular capacity.

3 Tesla Magnetic Resonance Imaging of the Nasal Cavities, Paranasal Sinuses and Adjacent Anatomical Structures in 13 Healthy Horses

J. Kaminsky, A. Bienert-Zeit, M. Hellige, B. Ohnesorge. Pferdeheilkunde 2014; 30(4): 413-431

The nasal cavities and paranasal sinuses of 13 healthy horses of different breeds aged 4 to 20 years were examined under general anaesthesia using 3 Tesla magnetic resonance imaging (MRI). Horses were positioned in dorsal recumbency. T2-weighted images were obtained in a transverse and dorsal orientation as well as T1-weighted images and proton density weighted images in a transverse orientation. Images were examined for the visualization of the nasal cavities, paranasal sinuses and adjacent anatomical structures. Differences and similarities in the appearance of the anatomical structures in the different MRI sequences as well as inter- and intraindividual differences and similarities were documented. In four selected planes of the transverse oriented T2-weighted images, the thickness of the venous plexus of the nasal mucosa of the left and right side could be measured in 12 horses. Planes and measurement points were chosen by defined anatomical landmarks. Visualized anatomical structures were well delineated in 3 Tesla magnetic resonance images. Inter- and intraindividual differences were present in the appearance of the nasal septum, the venous plexus of the nasal mucosa, the infraorbital canal and other structures in the examined healthy horses. The thickness of the venous plexus of the nasal mucosa was measured with up to 25.5 mm lining the spiral lamella of the ventral concha and the nasal meatus were entirely occluded by the nasal mucosa in some horses. Knowledge of the physiological appearance of anatomical structures in 3 Tesla MRI is fundamental in the use of this imaging modality as a diagnostic instrument. Interindividual differences in the appearance of anatomical structures are present in healthy horses and therefore not to be interpreted as pathologies in clinical cases.

Improvement of Motion Correction During Scintigraphic Examination of the Equine Thoracic and Lumbar Spine in Standing Horses

A. Sporn, D. Berner, W. Brehm, K. Winter, M. Mageed, M. Studt, K. Gerlach. Pferdeheilkunde 2014; 30(1): 91-97

Image quality of equine bone scintigrams of the thoracic spine is negatively affected by the continuous, slightly swaying movements of the standing sedated horse. In this study scintigraphic images of the thoracic spine of horses without (group 1) and with two radioactive markers (group 2) were investigated. Images were taken two, four and six hours (2h, 4h, 6h) after administration of 99mTc-HDP. After movement correction eight regions of interests (ROIs) were drawn in the images, four in the spinous processes and four in the adjacent soft tissue. The bone and soft-tissue uptake were determined and compared between the groups and the different time points. Afterwards computerized image analysis was used to define the contrast via bone to soft-tissue ratio as a measure of image quality. The bone to soft-tissue ratio was significantly higher in group 2 than in group 1 at every time point after injection (2h: $p = 0.001$; 4h: $p = 0.006$; 6h: $p = 0.009$). Bone scintigrams acquired with radioactive markers result in better summation images. Therefore, it is recommended to investigate the thoracic and lumbar spine in the standing sedated horse with additional radioactive markers.

Diagnostic of Pulmonary Abscesses in Foals – Comparison of Sonographic and Radiographic Examination

M. Venner, S.M. Walther, B. Münzer, P. Stadler. Pferdeheilkunde 2014; 30(5): 561-566

The aim of this study was to evaluate the diagnostic value of sonographic and radiographic examination in an early state of abscess-forming pneumonia in foals. Clinical and haematological examination as well as thoracic sonography and radiography was performed on 61 foals on a Warmblood stud. Nineteen foals were healthy and showed no clinical, no haematological and no sonographic signs of pneumonia. Fourty-two foals were clinically suspicious of pneumonia or showed a leukocytosis and had at least one pulmonary abscess at sonography. Altogether, 90 abscesses were detected sonographically in the 42 sick foals. Two chest radiographs (X-ray beam right to left and left to right) were taken of each foal and evaluated by three experienced equine internists blinded to the clinical findings of the foals. The number and location of abscesses were documented. A discrepancy was noted in the findings of the radiographs for signs of abscesses between the observers. Radiographic evaluation revealed an abscessing pneumonia in only 20 of the 42 sick foals. The location of the abscesses revealed at sonography and radiology agreed in only 21 abscesses. Finally a good match between radiologic and sonographic findings of abscesses was assessed in the area restricted to the central region of the lung. The results indicate that thoracic radiography is less reliable under field conditions compared to sonography. Sonography seemed to be more sensitive for the diagnosis of pulmonary abscesses in foals.